Chest X-ray Interpretation
for Radiographers, Nurses and Allied Health Professionals

For the full range of M&K Publishing books please visit our website:
www.mkupdate.co.uk

Chest X-ray Interpretation
for Radiographers, Nurses and Allied Health Professionals

Karen Sakthivel-Wainford
HDCR(R), MSc, PgCert
Advanced Radiographer Practitioner, Leeds General Infirmary

Chest X-ray Interpretation for Radiographers, Nurses and Allied Health Professionals

Karen Sakthivel-Wainford

ISBN: 978-1-910451-27-4

First published 2019

All rights reserved. No part of this publication may be reproduced, stored in a retrieval system, or transmitted in any form or by any means, electronic, mechanical, photocopying, recording or otherwise, without either the prior permission of the publishers or a licence permitting restricted copying in the United Kingdom issued by the Copyright Licensing Agency, 90 Tottenham Court Road, London, W1T 4LP. Permissions may be sought directly from M&K Publishing, phone: 01768 773030, fax: 01768 781099 or email: publishing@mkupdate.co.uk

Any person who does any unauthorised act in relation to this publication may be liable to criminal prosecution and civil claims for damages.

British Library Cataloguing in Publication Data

A catalogue record for this book is available from the British Library

Notice

Clinical practice and medical knowledge constantly evolve. Standard safety precautions must be followed, but, as knowledge is broadened by research, changes in practice, treatment and drug therapy may become necessary or appropriate. Readers must check the most current product information provided by the manufacturer of each drug to be administered and verify the dosages and correct administration, as well as contraindications. It is the responsibility of the practitioner, utilising the experience and knowledge of the patient, to determine dosages and the best treatment for each individual patient. Any brands mentioned in this book are as examples only and are not endorsed by the publisher. Neither the publisher nor the authors assume any liability for any injury and/or damage to persons or property arising from this publication.

To contact M&K Publishing write to:

M&K Update Ltd · The Old Bakery · St. John's Street

Keswick · Cumbria CA12 5AS

Tel: 01768 773030 · Fax: 01768 781099

publishing@mkupdate.co.uk

www.mkupdate.co.uk

Designed and typeset by Mary Blood

Printed in Scotland by Bell & Bain, Glasgow

Contents

Introduction *vii*

Acknowledgements *viii*

1. The radiographs and anatomy of the chest x-ray *1*
2. A systematic approach to reviewing the chest image *13*
3. Felson's silhouette sign *15*
4. Consolidation and collapse *19*
5. Overview of cardiovascular disorders and heart failure *27*
6. Lung tumours *33*
7. Lung nodules *43*
8. Chest trauma *49*
9. Tubes, lines and pacemakers *55*
10. Chronic chest conditions *63*
11. Tuberculosis *69*
12. 60 cases *75*

References and further reading *197*

Index *201*

Introduction

I have been reporting musculoskeletal radiographs for more than 20 years. However, radiographers in the Leeds Trust only started reporting chest x-rays five years ago. I and a colleague, being the first two to do this, duly set off for the reporting course at Bradford University with much trepidation (well, I did, really). As the university course progressed, along with our in-house learning, there was even more to learn than I had anticipated. How can one x-ray (two, if you are lucky enough to have a lateral view) be so complicated? I think this last statement will ring true for many who review chest x-rays. They are the most difficult plain film to report.

During this training process, I found few books on chest reporting that suited my initial needs. At the beginning of the course, I wanted a reasonably simple text that introduced me to the basics. There were a few books that did this, but I also wanted lots of different cases, with radiographs that I could actually see, so this is the gap that this book attempts to fill.

We begin with the anatomy of the chest x-ray, as visualised on the posterior anterior (PA) and lateral images. (When I teach reporting, I always say that you need to start with the normal anatomy, so that you know what is abnormal.) This is followed by a short chapter on having a systematic approach when reporting chest x-rays, then the silhouette sign as described by Felson, then chapters on consolidation and collapse, heart failure, tumours, lung nodules, chest trauma, tubes, lines and pacemakers, chronic chest conditions and tuberculosis. These chapters are followed by a final chapter that includes 60 cases for you to review.

In order to ensure complete anonymity, any clinical details given may not be the actual ones, but they are still appropriate to the image. In the process of removing names, some markers may also have been removed.

Today, many other healthcare professionals (besides Radiographers, Radiologists and other medics) are involved in reviewing chest x-rays. This book will therefore be useful for advanced nurse practitioners, A&E practitioners and major trauma practitioners, as well as radiographers, trainee reporting radiographers plus junior medics. However, it should always accompany a training course. For more details on the conditions discussed, please refer to detailed reference books and your Consultant Radiology colleagues.

This book is a good starting point in reviewing chest x-rays, and I hope it will encourage you to read and learn more about the 'complicated' chest x-ray image.

Acknowledgements

Thanks, firstly, to the Chest Consultant Radiologists at the Leeds General Infirmary, Dr Mike Darby and Dr Shishir Karthik, for teaching, supporting and mentoring my colleague and me through the chest reporting course, and their continuing support and assistance. Secondly, to Paul Atkinson, my long-time colleague and friend, for use of some of his references and some cases from the Bradford University course.

Thanks also to: Gill Roe for use of her images from the NG tube assessment; to the radiology department of the Leeds General Infirmary (as well as other hospital radiology departments in the Leeds Trust) for their continued support and use of their radiographs in this book. To Bradford University, for their chest reporting course and allowing me to use some of the work I did on their course in this book.

Last, but not least, thanks to my husband for his ongoing support and computer expertise, and to my family both in the UK and India.

THE RADIOGRAPHS AND ANATOMY OF THE CHEST X-RAY

Posterior anterior x-rays

The chest x-ray is normally taken PA (posterior anterior) standing, when the patient's condition permits, at a distance of 180cm, the scapula rotated away from the lungs, centred at thoracic vertebra 4 (T4) on full inspiration (as demonstrated below). However, some centres suggest centring at T4, then angling the x-ray tube to T6 to avoid irradiating the sensitive eyes. X-raying the chest PA and at 180cm reduces magnification of the heart. Removing the scapula from the lungs avoids misinterpretation of the overlying scapula as pathology. It also allows clear visualisation of the lungs. Poor inspiration will make the heart look larger, and may give the appearance of basal shadowing and cause the trachea to appear deviated to the right. If the patient is standing, it is easier for them to take a deep breath in.

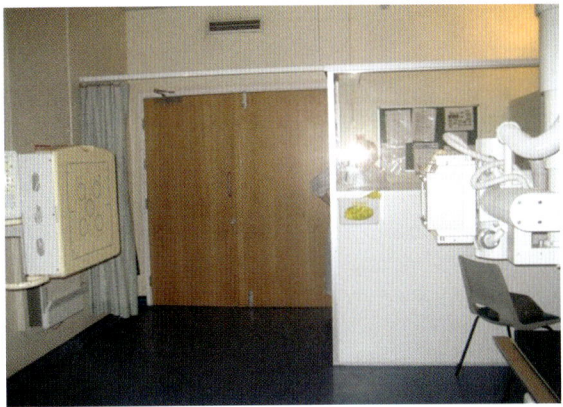

Figure 1.1: The X-ray room with digital wall stand

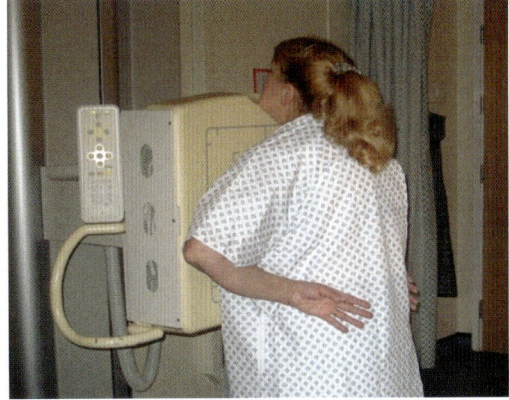

Figure 1.2: X-raying a PA chest

When reviewing the chest image, the first thing to check (before the anatomy or anything else) is whether the correct patient has been x-rayed on the correct date. Having checked these details, you can then assess the quality of the image, as this may affect your final interpretation.

Table 1.1: Quality issues

Issue	
PA, AP, sitting or supine	This will affect magnification/heart size
Rotation	Medial ends of clavicles should be equidistant from spinous process of vertebra
Lordotic/kyphotic	Clavicles should be posterior end of 4th rib, not above or below
Scapula removed from lungs	If not, be careful with interpretation
Full inspiration	Inspired to 5–6.5 anterior ribs, or 10/11 posterior ribs
Entire lungs included on image	If not, repeat may be required
Artefacts	Beware that an artefact is not misinterpreted as pathology
Correct marker/annotations	Is the patient really dextracardia?

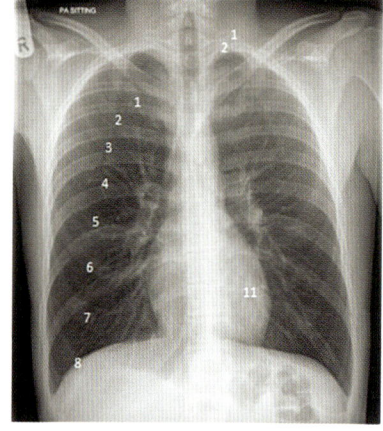

Anterior ribs being counted at this side

Posterior ribs being counted at this side

Figure 1.3: Counting ribs

If assessing inspiration, we first need to know which ribs we are counting – anterior or posterior. The above image demonstrates this. In certain conditions the lungs will be hyperventilated, and more than 11 posterior ribs will be visualised. In emphysema, the lungs may be so hyper-inflated that the diaphragm is flattened. The height of the diaphragm should normally be 1.5cm (see Figure 1.4, which shows how the diaphragm is measured).

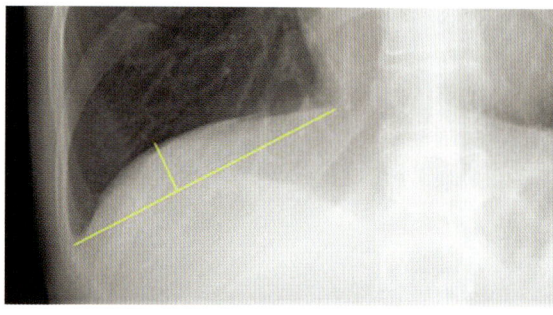

Figure 1.4: Measuring the height of the diaphragm, which is normally 1.5cm

If the patient is rotated, this will affect how the mediastinum is projected. Rotation to the right on a PA chest x-ray will result in the superior vena cava and/or other vessels arising from the arch of the aorta becoming more prominent. Severe rotation may result in one lung appearing darker than the other, giving a false impression of some underlying pathology.

A lordotic chest x-ray makes it difficult to accurately assess the pathology of the bases next to the diaphragm. The bases may become ill defined, mimicking pathology, and/or abdominal structures may be projected over the diaphragm and bases. A kyphotic image is most often produced when the patient is kyphotic due to vertebral collapse.

Obtaining a perfect-quality chest x-ray is difficult and the patient's condition may sometimes make it impossible. You will therefore often have to review a less than perfect-quality chest x-ray. Do this with caution, remembering the effects that rotation, poor inspiration and other factors may have on the final image. In most cases, it is still possible to answer the clinical question. However, if you have any doubt, a repeat x-ray (often when the patient is more able to cooperate), a lateral view (if possible), or further imaging may be required.

The patient's condition may often prohibit a PA image. In this case, the patient may have to be x-rayed anterior posterior (AP) in a chair, trolley or bed, or even supine. This will result in increased magnification of the heart and mediastinal structures. An AP sitting image is still taken at a distance of 180cm. However, a supine image is often taken at much less – around 140–120 cm, depending on the x-ray equipment, and how low the trolley or bed can go.

The AP sitting image may be lordotic. If so, take this into consideration when reviewing. Remember also, with a supine patient, fluid within the lungs will tend to sink to the posterior lungs, whereas air will rise. Likewise, effusions and a pneumothorax will appear differently in a supine patient compared to an erect patient (for more on this, see pp. 51–2). In both patient types, increased magnification makes it difficult to accurately assess the mediastinum.

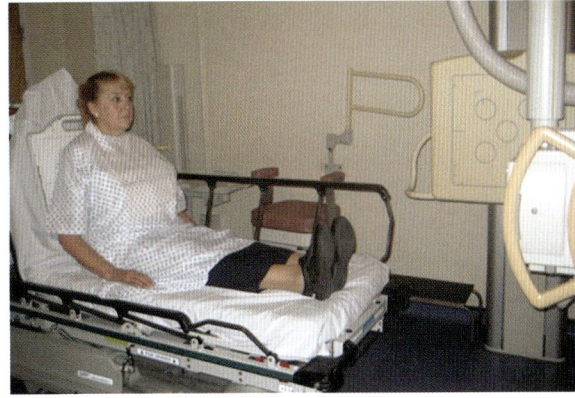

Figure 1.5: AP sitting chest x-ray (slightly lordotic, requiring angulation of x-ray tube)

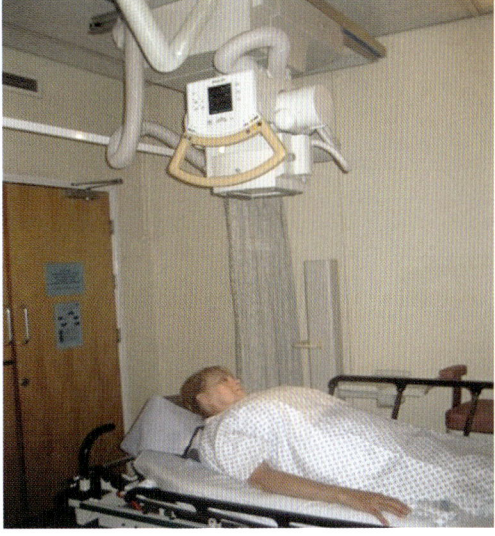

Figure 1.6: Supine chest x-ray

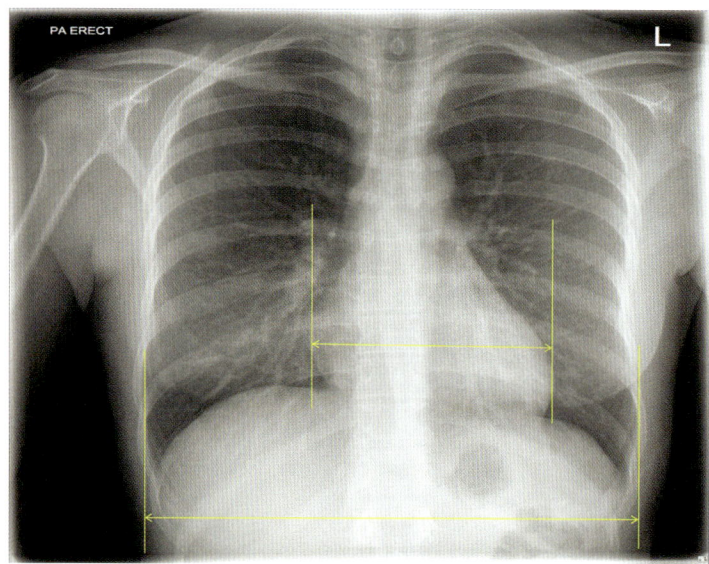

Figure 1.7 Measuring the heart size

The cardiothoracic ratio (CTR) in a PA patient is normally 50%, whereas on an AP sitting or supine image 60% is a good guideline. Please see Figure 1.7 for guidance on measuring CTR.

PA/AP/supine x-rays

Now we move on to the anatomy demonstrated on a PA/AP/supine chest x-ray. The basic anatomy is best visualised on a labelled chest radiograph.

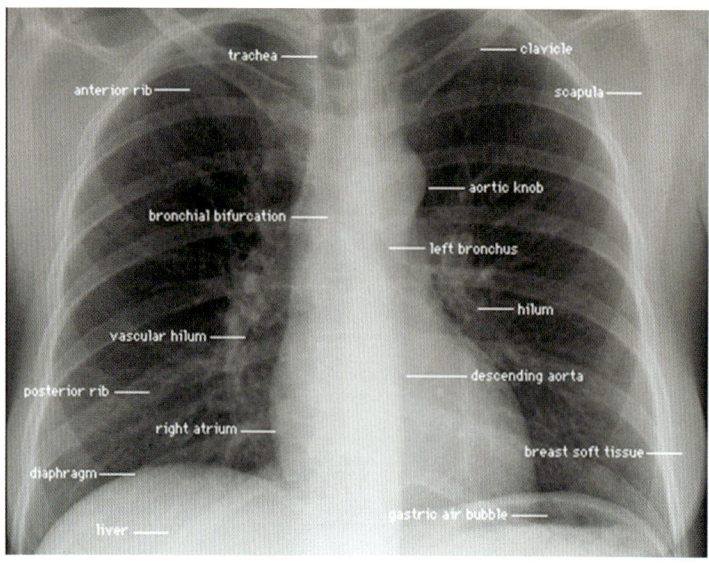

Figure 1.8 Know your chest anatomy

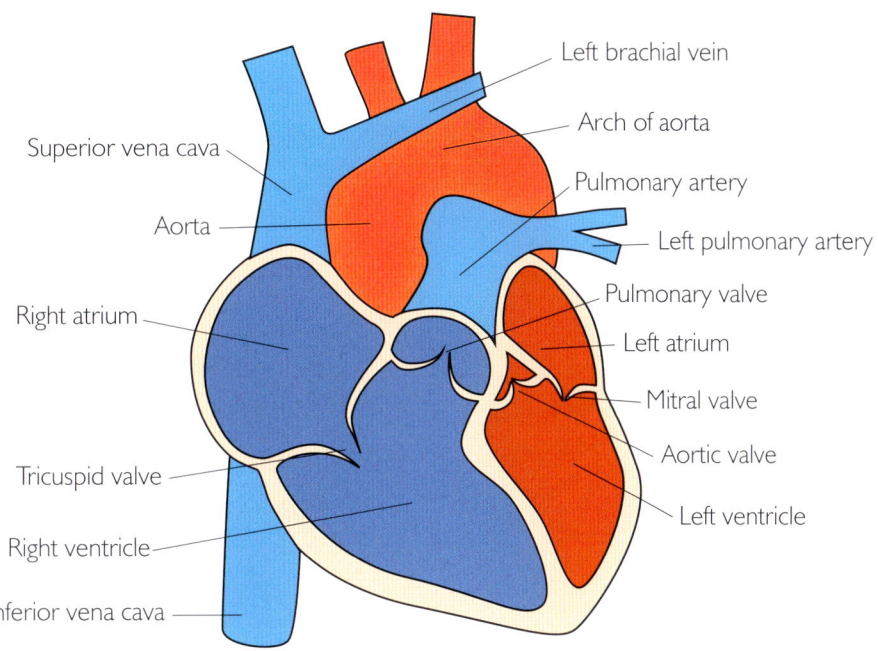

Figure 1.9 The heart structures on the chest x-ray

There are several other anatomical structures you need to know about when reviewing/reporting chest x-rays. The diaphragms, as previously mentioned, may be flattened in the hyperventilated chest. However, the right diaphragm is normally 1–2cm higher than the left, as demonstrated in Figure 1.10 below.

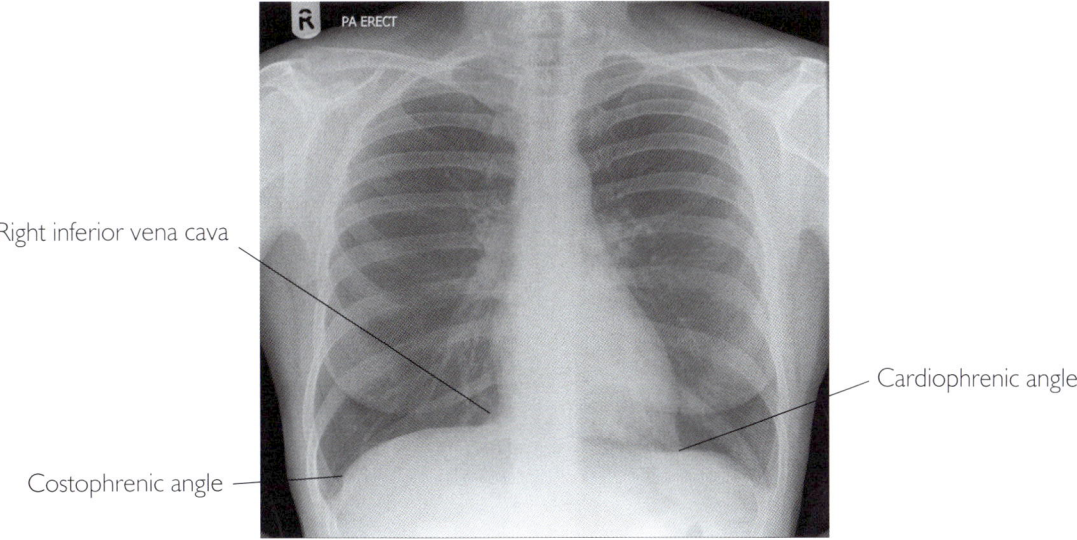

Figure 1.10 The diaphragms

The right lung has three lobes: the right upper lobe (RUL), the right middle lobe (RML), and the right lower lobe (RLL) as demonstrated in Figure 1.11. Meanwhile, the left lung has two lobes: the left upper lobe (LUL) and the left lower lobe (LLL), and also has the lingula. Figure 1.11 shows how little of the posterior base of the lungs is demonstrated on the frontal chest radiograph.

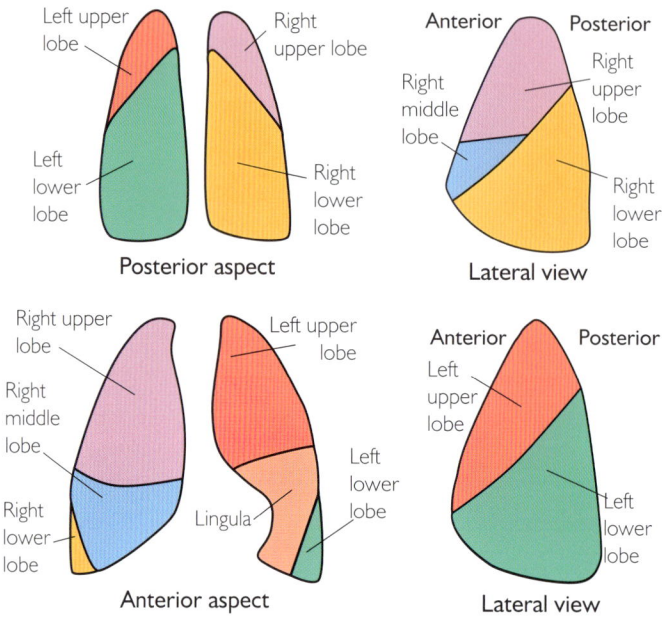

Figure 1.11 The lobes of the lungs

However, when describing the chest x-ray in a report, it is more common to divide the lungs into zones as demonstrated in Figure 1.12.

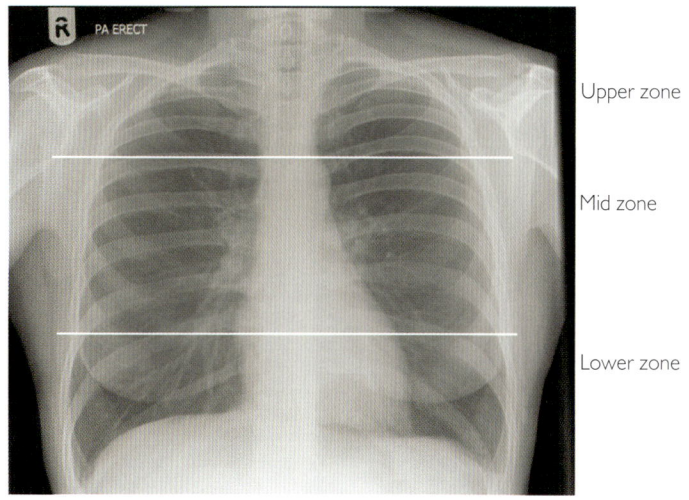

Figure 1.12 Zones on the chest x-ray

Displacement of the fissures on a chest x-ray may be due to collapse or mass so you should always try to visualise these. The middle fissure should lie around the 6th posterior rib.

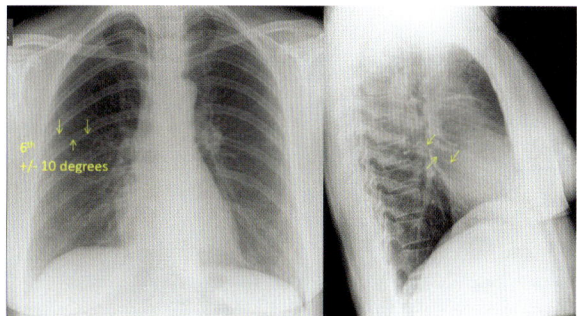

Figure 1.13 Lung x-ray showing fissures

There are several mediastinal lines that should be reviewed on a frontal radiograph, although they are often difficult (and sometimes impossible) to visualise. These include the:
- Anterior junction line: where the lungs meet anteriorly, not present above the sternal notch
- Posterior junction line: where the lungs meet posteriorly, seen superior to the sternal notch
- Right paratracheal stripe: normally up to 5mm with a bulge inferiorly where the azygos vein crosses the right main bronchus.

Bulging or widening of any of these lines may be a sign of a mediastinal mass.

Paravertebral stripe displacement is something else that should be reviewed. A left-sided thoracic vertebral stripe is normally visualised on the PA chest image. It is a deflection of the pleura posteriorly by the descending aorta, and it extends from the arch of the aorta to the diaphragm. Bulging of the left paravertebral stripe is consistent with pathology, the most common cause being haematoma following trauma/fracture of the thoracic spine. Alternatively, it may be caused by tumour or infection of the spine.

The right paravertebral stripe is not normally seen until older age when osteophytes cause displacement of the pleura; if seen in younger patients, there is some pathology present.

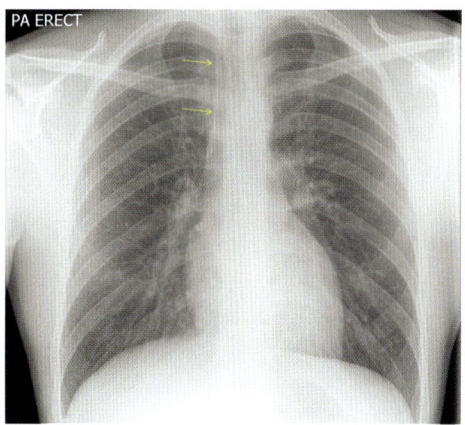

Figure 1.14 Right paratracheal stripe

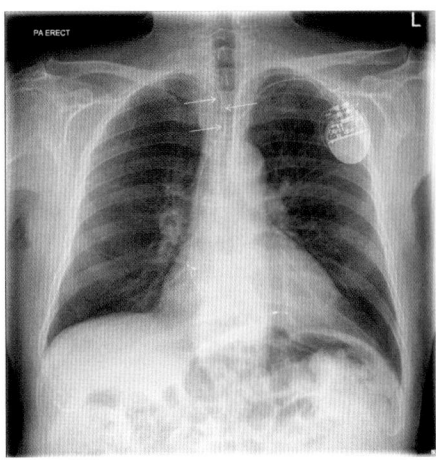

Figure 1.15 Anterior junction line

When reviewing the chest x-ray, you need to assess where the hilar are. Look for the hilar point in both lungs, as shown in Figure 1.16. The left hilum should be at the same level or higher than the right, never lower. The hilar density on each side should be similar. The hilar shadows are almost entirely due to the pulmonary arteries and veins. Air in the major bronchi can be visualised, but their walls are not usually visible.

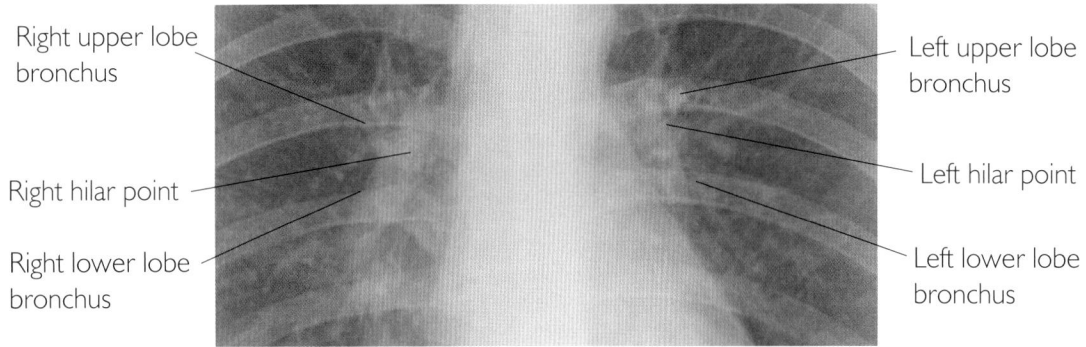

1.16 The hilar

Most Trusts in the UK rarely take lateral chest x-ray images. In fact at a recent study day I heard a radiologist say, 'No one takes lateral views as they don't know what they are looking at.' Surely this is a training issue?

In the large Leeds Trust where I work, a lateral chest x-ray is taken on GP patients over 55 years of age. If there is an area of suspicion on the PA radiograph, a lateral image will be taken by the examining radiographer. The radiation dose of a lateral chest x-ray is much lower than that of a CT (computerised tomography) scan; and when there is an area of suspicion on the PA image, taking a lateral radiograph may immediately answer the clinical question without resorting to CT. For instance, the lateral chest x-ray may demonstrate that the area of suspicion on the PA image is in fact a composite shadow, pericardial fat pad or artefact.

Though a CT may still sometimes be required (e.g. to investigate a mass), a lateral chest x-ray often clarifies questionable abnormalities. For instance, the GP patient over the age of 55 with a cough is often having a chest x-ray not only to look for consolidation but to assess for lung cancer. In this case, the addition of a lateral radiograph gives much more information, indeed the tumour on occasions may only be identified on the lateral radiograph. Feigin (2010), in his paper 'Lateral chest x-ray; a systematic approach', agrees that the lateral chest x-ray 'is valuable; and should be thought of as a full half of the routine chest radiograph'. He says, 'The lateral often provides key findings that are not visible on the frontal'.

Remember, when reviewing the PA image, some of the lungs are not visualised. The posterior/inferior sections are only visualised on the lateral chest image. In fact, when reviewing a PA image, I have seen a mass demonstrated below the diaphragm, but when reviewing the lateral I saw that it was within the lungs at the posterior base. The hilar are also often more easily visualised on the lateral view, where they are free from overlying structures.

Lateral x-rays

We will now look at reviewing the lateral chest image.

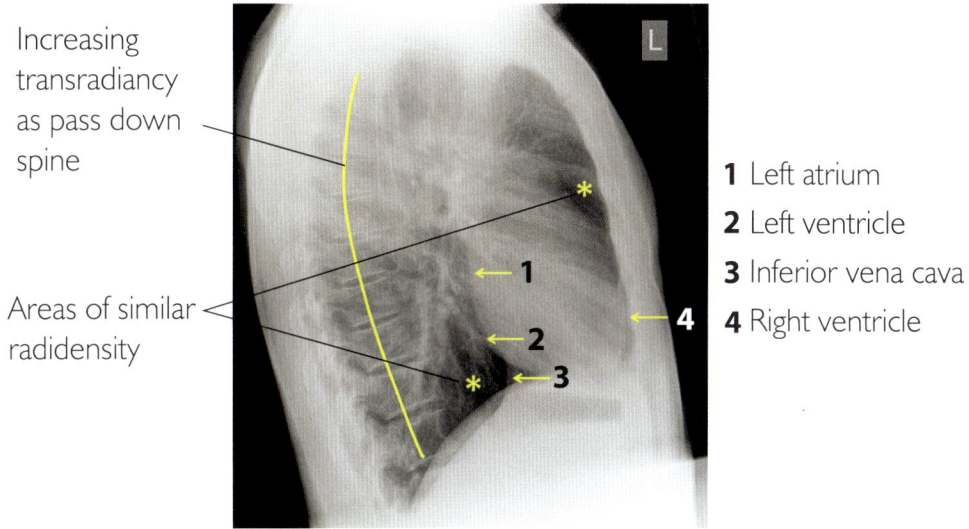

Figure 1.17 The lateral chest x-ray

The density of the upper retrosternal and retrocardiac (1 and 2, in the above diagram) should be of equal radiolucency. If this is not the case, this raises suspicion of a mass, which may be consolidation but could also be an anterior mediastinal mass, such as lymphoma. As you review the thoracic spine, there should be increasing transradiancy as you travel caudally because of the increased density of the shoulders. If the lungs over the lower thoracic spine are as dense as the upper, there is overlying pathology, which may indicate consolidation/mass or collapsed lung.

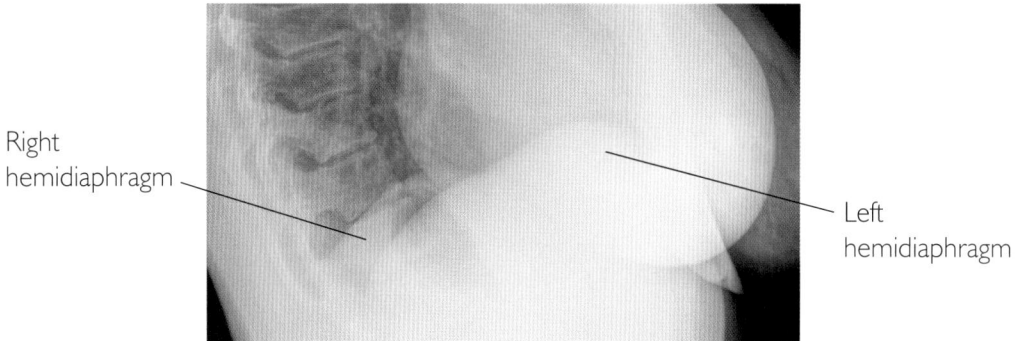

Figure 1.18 The diaphragms on the lateral view

The right diaphragm is easily identified on the lateral radiograph, as it is visualised as far as the anterior chest wall. The left diaphragm, however, is only visualised up to its junction with the heart. If either diaphragm is not clearly demonstrated, you should begin to consider overlying consolidation/mass or collapse at the lower lobe. Review the PA image to assess further.

Review the hilar area very carefully on the lateral image, as this is the area where lung nodules/masses may be visualised. The distal end of the left bronchus is visible as a round lucency, which is normally located near the apparent centre of the lungs. If there are two round lucencies in this area, the upper one is the right upper lobe bronchus and the lower one is the left main bronchus.

The opacities of the normal hilum are the two main pulmonary arteries as they enter the lungs. The bronchi follow the same path as the pulmonary arteries but are not visualised. All right pulmonary arteries are anterior and lateral to their respective bronchi. I am quite a visual person and recognise anatomy in musculoskeletal (MSK) reporting by shapes and appearance. I find the same applies to chest x-rays. The right pulmonary artery has a very white opacity, anterior to the airway in the centre, and has an ovoid appearance. The left pulmonary artery is less opaque and lies above the lucency of the left main bronchus. Its posterior margin curves inferior to the aorta with the same shape as the arch of the aorta.

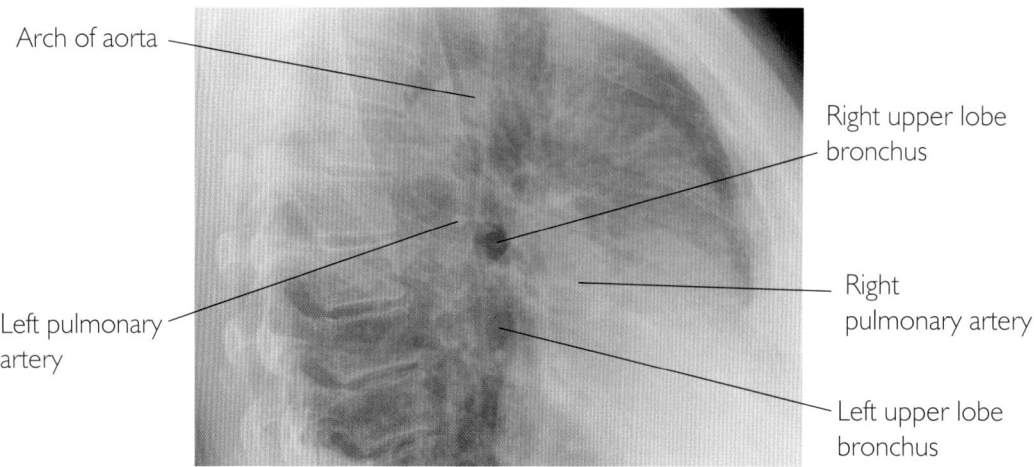

Figure 1.19 The hilar

Conclusion

This chapter has looked at the projections of the chest, and how the quality of the image may affect your review/report and the anatomy visualised. Another important aspect is to have a system when reviewing chest x-rays, and this is the subject of the next chapter.

Key points to remember

- *Is this the correct patient?*
- *Have you checked the clinical details and previous history?*
- *How was the patient x-rayed?*
- *Will the quality/position affect your interpretation and report?*
- *Look at previous images.*
- *Know your anatomy inside out.*

A SYSTEMATIC APPROACH TO REVIEWING THE CHEST IMAGE

When reviewing any x-ray image, you need a system, and this is even more important with the chest x-ray. Firstly, check that you are reviewing the correct patient's image, x-rayed on the correct date.

Then, very importantly with the chest, check previous images and review them, comparing them with the current image you are reviewing. Previous images will give you additional information that might not be included on the request card, such as a history of cancer or the fact that the patient has had a previous lobectomy. They will also allow you to assess whether a certain appearance is chronic or acute.

Next, you need to assess the quality of the image and consider whether it is going to affect your report/review.

Look at the clinical details – for instance, what is the clinician looking for, if it is cardiac failure? Of course, you should review everything on the images, but look especially carefully for signs that will answer the clinical question. For instance, state on the report whether or not cardiac failure is seen.

Now assess the radiograph in minute detail, magnifying and windowing as required. Review everything. It doesn't matter which system you use, as long as you have a system that includes everything, with special attention paid to the hidden areas behind the heart, the hilar, apices and bases. Don't forget to look at all the bones and joints and all the lines and other features mentioned in Chapter 1, as well as the cardiothoracic ratio.

The ABCDEF method is a useful way of remembering to review each of the areas in turn:

A – Apices and angles
B – Bases and bones
C – Cardiac (behind and within the heart)
D – Domes of diaphragm
E – Extra-thoracic
F – Foreign bodies (lines, tubes position)

Key points to remember

- *Check everything in minute detail.*
- *Window and magnify.*
- *Check lungs, heart, mediastinum, hilar and diaphragms.*
- *Check all anatomical lines mentioned in Chapter 1.*
- *Do not forget the bones and joints.*
- *Use the ABCDEF system.*
- *Check for inserted lines – are they in the correct position?*
- *Relate findings to clinical details.*

FELSON'S SILHOUETTE SIGN

What is the silhouette sign?

The silhouette sign gets its name from the fact that an intrathoracic radiopacity, if in anatomical contact with a border of the heart, diaphragm or aorta, will obscure that border. The first reference to it was made in around 1935, by Dr H. Kennon Dunham of Cincinnati, who often stated that obliteration of the left border of the heart by a contiguous pulmonary density indicated disease of the lingula. Interestingly a similar finding on the right was never mentioned (Felson 1973a). But it was Ben Felson, a twentieth-century American radiologist, who first fully described the silhouette sign in 1950, and continued to research its uses for the next 20 years, documenting his findings in his many chest radiology books.

Felson's first experiments in this field involved using an x-ray film carton filled with heated paraffin and waiting for it to solidify. This represented the heart, and air in another box represented the lungs; mineral oil was placed in a third carton to represent a diseased area of the lung. These were then placed in different positions and x-ray images taken. From these experiments, Felson hoped to find out how to localise an intrathoracic lesion on the posterior anterior radiograph.

One may wonder why, as a lateral radiograph would confirm the location of the lesion. However, there are many situations (e.g. when the patient is in intensive care, or being resuscitated) where a lateral view is not possible or practical. Also, routine chest x-rays are often posterior anterior view only, so it is important to be able to identify and locate lesions on this one image, although one could always recall the patient for a lateral chest x-ray.

Today, if a lesion was found, a CT scan would be carried out, but Felson's experiments took place before chest CT was thought of. It is better, however, to obtain as much knowledge as possible concerning chest radiographs so that subtle findings are not missed. A quote from Felson himself best sums up the silhouette sign: 'the explanation of the silhouette sign rests on the fact that the delineation of any roentgen shadow depends partly on differences in radiographic density' (Felson & Felson 1950, Felson 1973a).

At this stage, it is useful to list some of the relative absorption values for different tissues for an image taken at 60kv, before we proceed to look at the uses of Felson's silhouette sign. (Note that chest x-rays today are taken at a higher kv value of 80.)

Relative absorption values of tissues for 60kv radiation
- Water 1.0
- Carbon 0.7
- Fat 0.5
- Air 0.0001

(Felson 1973a)

Uses of Felson's silhouette sign

The silhouette sign has two important applications. Firstly, it enables us to localise a shadow by observing which borders are lost. For instance, loss of the heart border must mean the shadow lies in the anterior half of the chest; alternatively, loss of part of the diaphragm outline indicates disease of the pleura or lower lobes.

Secondly, it enables us to diagnose disorders such as consolidation even when there is uncertainty as to the presence of an opacity. A wedge- or lens-shaped opacity may be difficult to see because of the way the shadow fades out at the edges, and a completely collapsed lobe may also be difficult to see; if these lesions are in contact with the mediastinum or diaphragm, it causes loss of their normal sharp boundaries.

To conclude, when examining the lungs on a normal chest x-ray, the silhouettes of the heart borders, the ascending and descending aorta, the aortic knob and the hemidiaphragms should be clear. Obliteration of any of these silhouettes can be caused by consolidation, mass, etc. However, all these structures are in contact with a specific portion of the lung. By determining which structure is obliterated, you can therefore determine where the lung pathology is located (Armstrong & Wastie 1989, Felson 1973a).

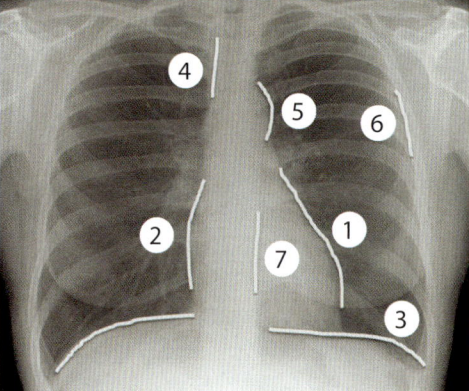

If there was increased shadowing with silhouette sign at the following interfaces, where would the pathology be located?

1 Left heart border: lingular disease
2 Right heart border: right middle lobe disease
3 Diaphragms: lower lobe pathology
4 Right paratracheal stripe: nodal disease
5 Aortic knuckle: anterior mediastinum or left upper lobe
6 Chest wall: lung/pleura/rib pathology
7 Paraspinal line: posterior thorax or posterior mediastinum

Figure 3.1 Silhouette sign – locating pathology

Areas where caution is needed when using the silhouette sign

Several journal articles and texts, in particular De Lacey and his colleagues in their book, *The Chest X-ray: A survival guide* (2008), suggest that caution is needed in some areas when using the silhouette sign. These are outlined below.

- Be careful when viewing an anterior posterior sitting or supine chest x-ray, as angulation cranially may project extra-pleural fat over the base of the left lung, resulting in loss of the left diaphragm.
- A large amount of fat may be situated between the pericardium, lung and dome of the diaphragm, which may blur the dome.
- A depressed sternum can produce loss of the right heart border
- In some patients, pulmonary vessels or fat are close to the heart border, resulting in blurring of the right heart border.

(De Lacey et al. 2008, Hollman et al. 1989, Reed 2003, Zylak 1988).

Felson's research and observations of other possible uses of the silhouette sign in the posterior anterior chest x-ray

Felson continued to observe and research uses of the silhouette sign and its principles. (The air bronchogram sign is explained in Chapter 4.) Bronchi are not normally demonstrated radiographically, but in an opacified lung they may be seen (Oktay 2011).

Felson observed that applying the silhouette sign to the border of the trachea is unreliable, as in many normal patients it cannot be seen; and the same applies to the cephalic aspect of the aortic knob. However, it can be applied to the right and left pulmonary arteries, as the lateral portion profiled by the lungs is visible on the posterior anterior chest x-ray.

The hilum convergence sign does not always work, as it requires a Bucky image and any obliquity makes it invalid, according to Felson (1973a). However, De Lacey *et al.* (2008) describe the hilum convergence sign and hilum overlay sign in detail, as useful so-called 'power tools' when reviewing chest radiographs. Today, highly detailed digital images of chest x-rays are found in most radiology departments. These are often taken with an incorporated grid and are equally useful (indeed better) than the Bucky images Felson (1973a) speaks about. With good-quality chest x-ray images, the hilum convergence sign and hilum overlay sign are useful when assessing the posterior anterior chest image, but treat these signs with caution when assessing a rotated image (again, you need to consider how the quality of the image may affect your final report).

What are the hilum convergence and overlay signs?

The hilum convergence sign allows an enlarged hilum that is due to enlarged pulmonary arteries to be distinguished from enlargement due to tumour. If the vessels appear to arise medial to the enlarged hilar, then it is a tumour. However, if the vessels arise from or converge directly onto the enlarged hilar shadow, then the pathology is vascular.

The hilum overlay sign helps us distinguish between cardiac enlargement and anterior mediastinal mass. If the hilum is lateral to the lateral border of the mass, there is cardiac enlargement; if the hilum is medial to the lateral border of the mass, it is a mediastinal mass.

The cervicothoracic sign is based on the fact that if a thoracic lesion is in contact with the soft tissues of the neck, its continuous border will be lost. The cephalic border of the anterior mediastinum ends at the clavicles, whereas the posterior border ends much higher. Hence a lesion above the clavicles on the frontal view must lie posteriorly and be entirely within the thorax. If anterior, the cervical soft tissues would have obscured it. Both Felson (1973a) and De Lacey *et al.* (2008) agree the cervicothoracic sign is useful when assessing the posterior anterior chest x-ray.

Since the abdominal structures are mainly of water density, a sharply marginated mediastinal mass seen through the diaphragm, on a chest or abdominal image, must lie in the thorax; this is the thoracoabdominal sign (Felson 1973a, Lacey *et al.* 2008, Oktay 2011).

Conclusion

The silhouette sign is an extremely useful tool when assessing the posterior anterior chest x-ray. When we fully understand its use, it can allow us to visualise subtle lesions/pathologies and locate them. There are only minor areas of caution required in its use, and its main principles can be applied in other areas.

To conclude, a positive silhouette sign is very helpful. However, a negative silhouette sign does not guarantee that a given lobe of the lung is disease-free because it may be partially aerated and therefore not cause a silhouette sign.

Interestingly, newer texts and journals add little information to the initial research Felson did on the silhouette sign in the 1950s and his continued work in this area over the following 20 years. It is therefore extremely useful to read Felson's research and textbooks on the silhouette sign to fully understand its use.

Key points to remember

- *'…the explanation of the silhouette sign rests on the fact that the delineation of any roentgen shadow depends partly on differences in radiographic density' (Felson 1950, Felson 1973a).*
- *Always use Felson's silhouette sign when reviewing the chest x-ray.*
- *Know and use the hilum convergence and overlay signs.*
- *Know the cervicothoracic sign and its use.*
- *Know the limitations of Felson's silhouette sign.*

CONSOLIDATION AND COLLAPSE

What is consolidation?

Consolidation is caused by fluid filling the smaller bronchi, bronchioles and alveoli. The nature of the fluid cannot be determined radiographically. It could be pus as in infection, water as in pulmonary oedema, haemorrhage as in trauma or some of the vasculitides, or malignant cells as in alveolar carcinoma. Consolidation shadowing can range from subtle patchy areas to widespread confluent shadows.

The hallmark of consolidation is the presence of air bronchograms, as described by Felson's silhouette sign. Pure consolidation shows no loss of volume, but consolidation is often accompanied by collapse.

Air bronchograms

Air is seen in the trachea and proximal bronchi in a normal chest because these are surrounded by the soft tissues of the mediastinum. The airways distal to the proximal segmental bronchi are thin walled and not normally visible. However, when the normally aerated pulmonary parenchyma is replaced by non-aerated tissue (as in consolidation), the bronchi and bronchioles become visible as branching linear lucencies, which are known as air bronchograms. The air bronchogram sign specifically indicates a lung parenchyma process, as distinct from a pleural or mediastinal process.

Consolidation of a whole lobe

Consolidation of a whole lobe is often diagnostic of bacterial pneumonia. It is one of the commonest causes of morbidity and mortality in the UK (Das & Howlett 2009). Lobar consolidation produces an opaque lobe, except for the presence of air bronchograms. As the consolidated lobe is airless, the fissure between it and the normal lung does not appear as a line, but as a clear-cut border to the opacity.

Using the silhouette sign, we know that the boundary between the affected lobe and the adjacent heart, mediastinum and diaphragm will be invisible; this allows us to locate the area of consolidation accurately on the posterior anterior view. A lateral chest x-ray, if possible, in what could potentially be an extremely ill patient, will confirm the locality of the consolidation. However, if the posterior anterior/anterior posterior (PA/AP) chest x-ray view gives enough information for the consolidation to be located (reasonably accurately), diagnosed and treated appropriately, why do a lateral radiograph? Performing a lateral radiograph will increase the radiation dose to the patient (albeit by a small amount), as well as potentially causing them discomfort. Yet it won't alter the management of the patient. This is an area where a lateral view is not helpful or required (Armstrong & Wastie 1989, De Lacey et al. 2008, Felson 1973b).

Streptococcus pneumoniae is the commonest cause of lobar pneumonia, usually affecting one lobe only, with little or no collapse. Other less common causes of lobar pneumonia include:

- Staphylococcus aureus – especially in children; 40 to 60% of children develop pneumatoceles; effusion and pneumothorax are common
- Klebsiella pneumonia – often multilobar
- Streptococcus pyogenes – mainly affects the lower lobes
- Tuberculosis – most common in primary tubercolosis; collapse is common; right lung is affected twice as often as the left (Chapman & Nakielny 1992).

Patchy consolidation

Patchy consolidation (for example, one or more patches of ill-defined shadowing) is usually due to infection or infarction, or (less commonly) contusion or allergy. When spherical in shape, consolidation may be difficult to distinguish from a lung tumour; but usually serial films over a short interval show change if the shadow is due to consolidation. The air bronchogram sign is helpful, since it is common in consolidation but rare in tumours. However, if there is any reason to suspect a lung tumour a high-resolution computed tomography (HRCT) scan should be done and an appropriate referral pathway followed (Armstrong & Wastie 1989, Clarke 2012, Corne et al. 1997, De Lacey et al. 2008, Felson 1973b).

De Lacey et al. (2008) suggest adopting a 6-week chest x-ray rule in patients who have chest x-ray evidence of pneumonia, who smoke or have clinical or radiological features that suggest there may be an underlying bronchial carcinoma. If the chest x-ray at 6 weeks (following treatment for the pneumonia etc.) is not clear and there are no worrying features and the patient is clinically well, he suggests a further chest x-ray at 4 weeks, to ascertain that clearing is continuing.

However, for all smokers over 40 years of age, who have any clinical features of lung cancer de Lacey suggests a CT and bronchoscopy. NICE guidelines also suggest a 6-week follow-up in patients over 50 with consolidation or collapse, to ensure resolution of appearances. If consolidation/collapse is not starting to resolve after appropriate treatment after this time period and in this age group, this raises suspicion of lung cancer.

In the Leeds Trust it is more likely that an HRCT would be arranged for any patient whose chest x-ray was not clear after 6 to 8 weeks. This is a more cautious route, so that potential bronchial carcinomas are diagnosed and treated sooner, and I believe many other UK Trusts have adopted this pathway.

In the more elderly patient with consolidation, an 8-week (rather than 6-week) follow-up should be considered, as these patients may take longer to recover.

Pulmonary collapse

Pulmonary collapse (loss of volume of a lung or lobe) is sometimes referred to as atelectasis, and can be associated with consolidation. Location of both collapse and consolidation on a PA/AP chest x-ray

may be obtained by the use of Felson's silhouette sign (see Chapter 3). Pulmonary collapse may be due to any of the following:
- Bronchial obstruction
- Pneumothorax or pleural effusion
- Fibrosis of a lobe, usually following tuberculosis
- Bronchiectasis
- Pulmonary embolus.

Collapse due to bronchial obstruction

This occurs because no air can get into the lungs to replace the air absorbed from the alveoli. The most common causes are (Armstrong & Wastie 1989, Davies et al. 1990, Sunderamoorthy et al. 2005):
- Intraluminal occlusion, such as a mucous plug postoperatively or in asthmatic patients, or it may be due to a foreign body
- Bronchial wall lesions, usually primary carcinoma; rarely, endobronchial tuberculosis or bronchial adenoma
- Invasion or compression by adjacent mass, such as malignant tumour or enlarged lymph nodes
- A wrongly placed endotracheal tube
- Inhalation of a foreign body.

When the lobe is not aerated, it will lose much of its volume and will collapse, resulting in increased shadowing of the collapsed lobe on the radiograph and movement of other structures (e.g. trachea, hilum, horizontal fissure) to take up some of the void left by the collapsed lobe. The silhouette sign is important in identifying a collapsed lung or lobe.

Consolidation often accompanies lobar collapse. Occasionally the loss of volume is so severe that, unless it is tangential to the x-ray beam, it may be difficult to see. The silhouette sign is very useful in this situation, as the mediastinal (or diaphragmatic) borders will be ill defined adjacent to the collapsed lobe. The silhouette sign also helps in identifying, from the chest x-ray, which lobe is collapsed. Collapse of the anteriorly located lobes (the upper and middle) will obliterate portions of the mediastinal and heart outlines, whereas collapse of the lower lobes obscures the outline of the adjacent diaphragm and descending aorta.

When a lobe collapses, other structures move to take up the space. The unobstructed lobe on the side of the collapse expands (compensatory emphysema), resulting in displacement of fissures and movement of the hilum towards the collapsed lobe. The fissure is seen as a well-defined boundary to the airless lobe. The mediastinum and diaphragm may move towards the collapsed lobe. CT shows lobar collapse very well and is a useful secondary investigation in some cases. If the whole of one lung has collapsed, the entire hemithorax is opaque and there is marked mediastinal and tracheal shift towards the collapsed lung (Armstrong & Wastie 1989, Clarke 2012, Corne et al. 1997, De Lacey et al. 2008, Felson 1973b).

Collapse due to lobar fibrosis or bronchiectasis

In both of these, a lobe may be reduced in volume, sometimes quite severely, but normally remains partially aerated.

Collapse due to pneumothorax or pleural effusion

In both of these, the cause of the collapse should be identifiable. With a pneumothorax, it is often located at the apices, but may be demonstrated basally; a sharp fine line should be identified with no lung markings demonstrated distal to it.

When examining elderly patients, be careful not to mistake a skin fold for a pneumothorax. With a pneumothorax lung markings will not be seen distal to the sharp fine line; with a skin fold markings will be seen distal to the skin fold. Also be careful of mistaking large bullae for a pneumothorax; in this case, there will be other signs of emphysema on the image. If a tension pneumothorax is identified, immediate treatment is required (i.e. a chest drain). Theoretically, a tension pneumothorax should never be seen on an x-ray image; it should be diagnosed and treated clinically first.

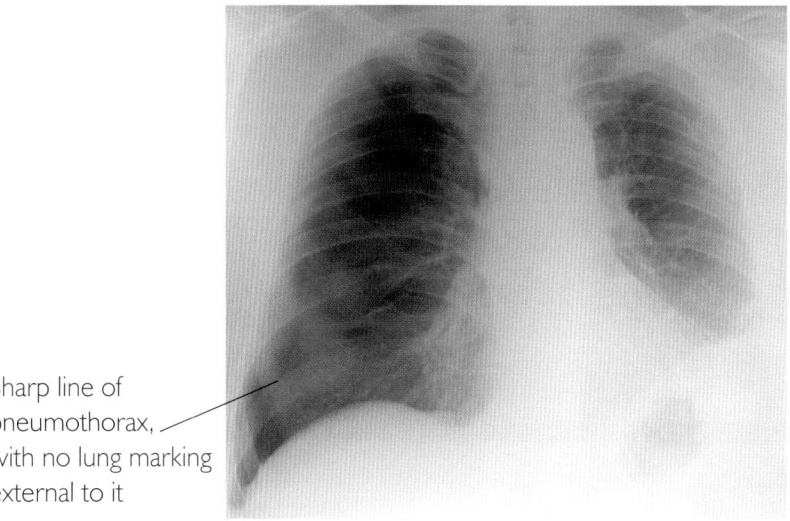

Sharp line of pneumothorax, with no lung marking external to it

Figure 4.1 Right-sided pneumothorax

Collapse due to pulmonary embolus

With this condition, the involved lobe or lobes usually show a combination of patchy consolidation and loss of volume (but often not much). However, a plain chest image cannot rule out pulmonary emboli. If a pulmonary embolus is suspected, vascular CT is often carried out (Armstrong & Wastie 1989).

Collapse of the lower left lobe

One area of collapsed lung field that requires extra caution when viewing the PA/AP chest x-ray is collapse of the left lower lobe. It is probably the easiest to miss, as the left lower lobe collapses down behind the heart. In this situation, the left lung field appears much darker than normal, and the heart shadow appears much whiter than normal. With careful observation, a white triangle can be seen behind the heart. The lateral radiograph, if taken, demonstrates a white triangle at the bottom posterior corner of the lung fields, and the vertebral bodies will appear whiter.

Examples of lobar collapse

Below are several examples of lobar collapse and how they are demonstrated on the x-ray image, using Felson's silhouette sign.

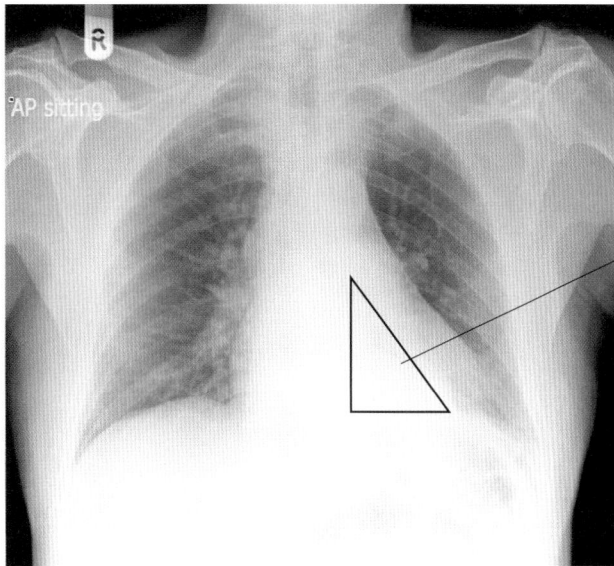

Figure 4.2 Sail sign of left lower lobe collapse (identified on the chest x-ray, investigated by CT)

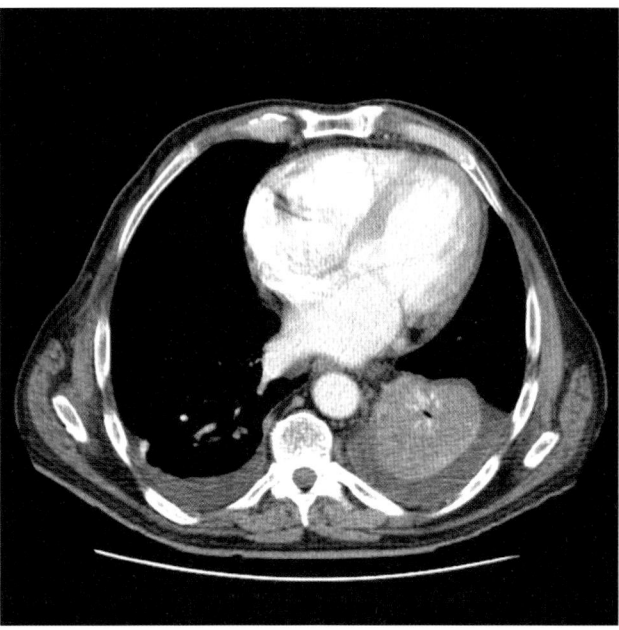

Figure 4.3 CT of left lower lobe collaps

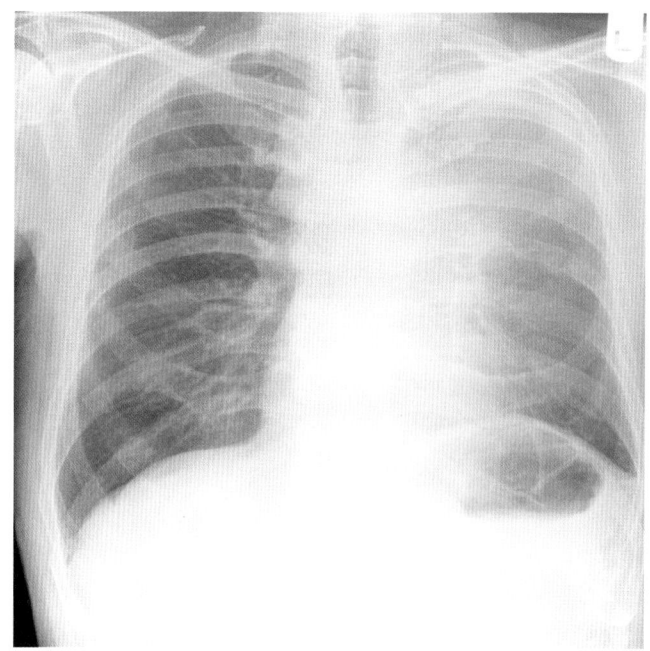

*Figure 4.4 Left upper lobe collapse
(gives a veil-like opacity, with loss of definition of the left heart border, consistent with Felson's silhouette sign)*

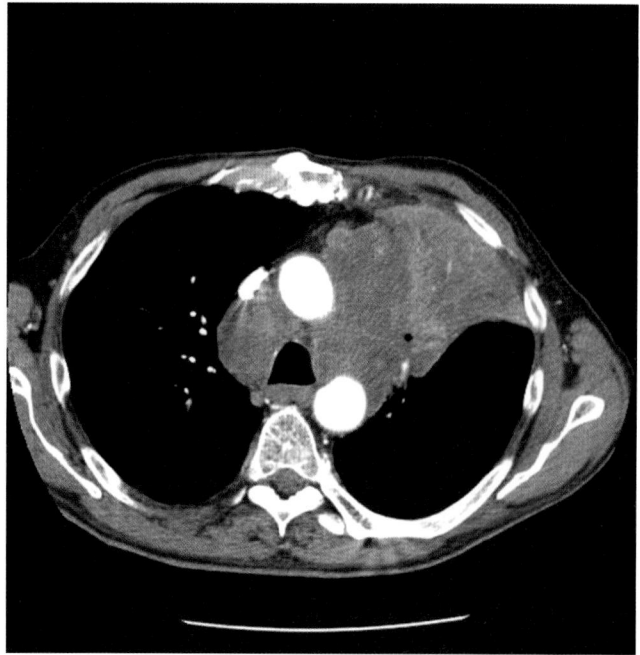

Figure 4.5 CT of left upper lobe collapse

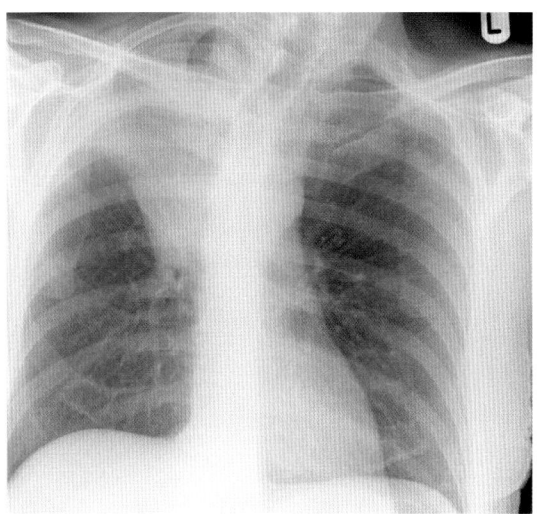

Figure 4.6 Right upper lobe collapse (using Felson's silhouette sign – loss of right upper mediastinal border)

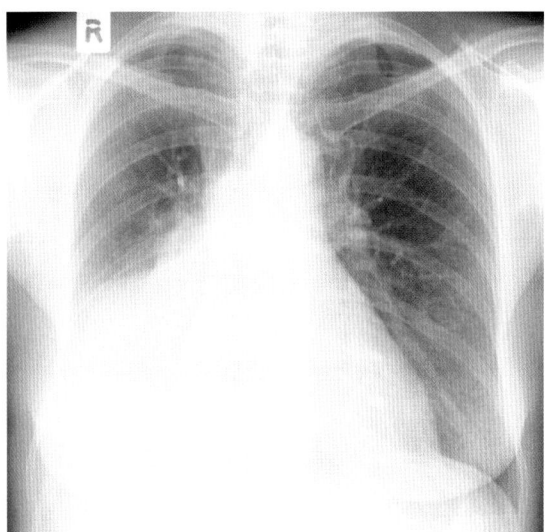

Figure 4.7 Right lower lobe collapse (using Felson's silhouette sign – loss of right diaphragmatic border)

De Lacey et al. (2008) describe various benign appearances that may be mistaken for lobar collapse. If in doubt, a lateral chest x-ray will confirm whether it is a benign appearance or not, and this will of course affect management of the patient. Below are some examples of benign appearances that may be mistaken for lobar collapse:

- Right upper lobe – be careful of the azygos fissure, and unfolded neck vessels, in the elderly
- Middle lobe – be careful of a depressed sternum, or fat touching the heart border
- Right lower lobe – be careful of epicardial fat pad, and the accessory fissure
- Left lower lobe – be careful of the unfolded aorta in the elderly, and a hiatus hernia
- Left upper lobe – no benign appearances requiring caution.

Conclusion

Collapse and consolidation may occur together or separately. Consolidation is a generic term; and if the cause of the consolidation is identifiable, this should be stated in the report. An air bronchogram may be seen in the consolidated area. Felson's silhouette sign is a useful tool for identifying the location of the collapse or consolidation on the PA/AP chest x-ray. Where there is any radiological or clinical suspicion that the collapse or consolidation is due to bronchial carcinoma, or any other carcinoma, then an HRCT should be performed, with appropriate referral.

Key points to remember

- *Know and use Felson's silhouette sign to identify consolidation and collapse.*
- *Be able to recognise the air bronchogram sign.*
- *If possible, assess and state cause of consolidation.*
- *Be able to identify different types of lobar collapse.*
- *Suggest follow-up 6–8 weeks in appropriate patients, as per NICE guidelines.*
- *Be able to distinguish pneumothorax from skin folds, bullae, etc.*

OVERVIEW OF CARDIOVASCULAR DISORDERS AND HEART FAILURE

Introduction

There are several clues to cardiovascular disorders on the chest x-ray, but only a few are specific enough to make a definitive diagnosis. Many patients will continue to have other diagnostic investigations, the most common being echocardiography, particularly when looking at valve function and chamber size. Other investigations may include angiography (to demonstrate the coronary arteries and other vessels), and in some centres magnetic resonance imaging (MRI).

This chapter will firstly look at identifying some of the clues to cardiac problems on the plain chest x-ray; and then briefly summarise some of the main cardiovascular disorders, identifying their possible appearance on the radiograph.

Signs of heart disease

Heart size

The cardiothoracic ratio (CTR) is a widely used but crude method of measurement (Armstrong & Wastie 1989). Most normal adult hearts have a CTR that does not exceed 50% when assessed on a posterior anterior erect chest x-ray on full inspiration. The observation of increasing heart size in comparison with previous images is often more useful than the CTR in isolation. De Lacey (2008) comments that the CTR in an individual can vary up to 0.5cm. This of course depends on rotation, position (PA versus AP, or supine), depth of inspiration, and whether the image is taken in diastole or systole. Another thing to be aware of is whether or not there is a cardiac fat pad – do not include this in the measurement of the heart.

Chamber hypertrophy and dilation

This is more accurately determined by an echocardiograph, which will determine whether enlargement is due to pericardial effusion or chamber enlargement. Diagnosing ventricular enlargement on chest x-rays is difficult, as only one or two of the borders of either ventricle will be visible. It is also difficult to distinguish ventricular hypertrophy from dilation. Often, all that can be determined is an increase in transverse cardiac diameter.

Assessing the atrial size on a chest x-ray is easier. The border of an enlarged left atrium is visible as a double contour within the right cardiac shadow. When dilated, the left atrial appendage is seen on the chest x-ray as a bulge below the main pulmonary artery; with gross enlargement, the left main bronchus is pushed superiorly. The posterior margin of the left atrium is best demonstrated on the lateral view. Right atrial enlargement causes an increase in the curvature of the right heart border.

Common causes of chamber enlargement

Armstrong and Wastie (1989) give a good summary of the common causes of chamber enlargement, as listed below.

Left atrial enlargement:
- Mitral stenosis
- Mitral incompetence
- Left atrial tumour, e.g. myxoma.

Right atrial enlargement:
- Right ventricle failure
- Tricuspid stenosis
- Tricuspid incompetence.

Left ventricular enlargement:
- Aortic and mitral incompetence
- Aortic stenosis
- Ischaemic heart disease and cardiomyopathy
- Patent ductus arteriosus and ventricular septal defects in cases with left to right shunts.

Right ventricular enlargements:
- Atrial septal defect
- Tricuspid regurgitation
- Pulmonary stenosis and pulmonary hypertension.

Pericardial disease

Chest x-ray is not the modality to diagnose a pericardial effusion. A patient may have life-threatening pericardial effusion and only mild cardiac enlargement. However, a marked increase or decrease in the cardiac diameter within 2 weeks is diagnostic of pericardial effusion.

Pericardial calcification is seen in approximately 50% of patients with constrictive pericarditis. It is usually post-infective in aetiology – tuberculosis and Coxsackie infections being the most common precursors (Armstrong & Wastie 1989, Ketai *et al.* 2006, Weissleder *et al.* 1997).

Pulmonary vessels

It is possible on the chest x-ray to assess the pulmonary artery for enlargement by looking at its degree of bulging. At the hilar, the right lower lobe artery can be measured; it should be between 9 and 16mm. The size of the vessels within the lungs reflects pulmonary blood flow. By observing the size of these vessels, it may be possible to diagnose increased pulmonary blood flow, decreased pulmonary blood flow, and pulmonary artery and pulmonary venous hypertension.

Increased pulmonary blood flow
Atrial septal defect, ventral septal defect and patent ductus arteriosus are common causes of blood being shunted from the systemic to the pulmonary circuits, thus increasing blood flow. In patients with severe left to right shunts, all the vessels from the main pulmonary artery to the periphery of the lungs are large; this is sometimes called pulmonary plethora.

Decreased pulmonary blood flow
To be recognised on a chest x-ray, the decrease in blood flow has to be substantial. When the pulmonary vessels are all small, it is known as pulmonary oligaemia. The commonest cause is Tetralogy of Fallot.

Pulmonary artery hypertension
The pressure in the pulmonary artery depends on cardiac output and pulmonary vascular resistance. The conditions that lead to significant pulmonary arterial hypertension tend to increase the resistance of blood flow through the lungs. Many lung conditions can result in this, as can pulmonary emboli and pulmonary arterial narrowing as a result of mitral disease. Pulmonary arterial hypertension has to be severe before it can be diagnosed on a chest x-ray.

The chest x-ray findings will be enlargement of the pulmonary artery and hilar arteries, the vessels within the lungs being normal or small. De Lacey et al. (2008) list some of the causes of pulmonary artery hypertension as: longstanding pulmonary venous hypertension, left to right shunts, pulmonary embolism, respiratory disease, high altitude, drugs and poison.

Pulmonary venous hypertension
Mitral valve disease and left ventricular failure are the commonest causes of pulmonary venous hypertension. In raised pulmonary venous pressure, in an upright patient, the upper zone vessels enlarge and in severe cases become larger than those in the lower zone (Armstrong & Wastie 1989, Chapman & Nakielny 1992, De Lacey et al. 2008, Ketai et al. 2006).

Pulmonary oedema
The commonest cardiac conditions causing pulmonary oedema are left ventricular failure and mitral stenosis. Cardiogenic pulmonary oedema occurs when the pulmonary venous pressure rises above 24mmHg. Initially the oedema is in the interstitial tissues of the lung, but as it becomes more severe, fluid collects in the alveoli. Both interstitial and alveoli pulmonary oedema can be recognised on plain chest x-rays.

Interstitial oedema
There are septa in the lungs that are invisible on a chest x-ray, because they consist only of a sheet of connective tissue. However, when these are thickened by oedema, the peripherally located septa may be seen as line shadows. These are called Kerley B lines; they are horizontal lines seen in the lower zones, never more than 2cm long. These lines reach the lung edge, which distinguishes them from blood vessels which never extend into the outer centimetre of lung. Other septa (known as Kerley A lines) radiate towards the hila or mid and upper zones. These are much thinner than the adjacent blood vessels, and normally 3–4cm in length. Another sign of interstitial oedema is that the outline of blood vessels may be seen, due to oedema collecting around them.

Alveolar oedema

This is a more severe form of oedema where the fluid collects in the alveoli. It is normally bilateral when it occurs, involving all the lobes. Shadowing is maximal close to the hila. This pattern of oedema is sometimes referred to as 'butterfly' or 'bat's wing' pattern (Armstrong & Wastie 1989, Chapman & Nakielny 1992, De Lacey et al. 2008, Ketai et al. 2006).

Cardiac disorders

Heart failure

One or all of the following signs may be seen on a chest x-ray:
- Cardiac enlargement
- Raised pulmonary venous pressure, i.e. enlargement of the vessels in the upper zones of the lung
- Evidence of pulmonary oedema
- Pleural effusions, usually bilateral, but if unilateral more often on the right side.

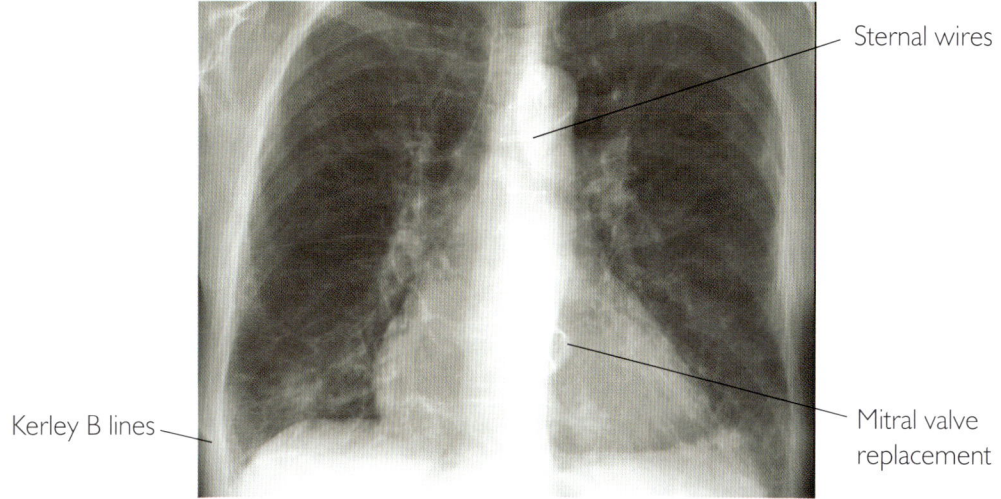

Figure 5.1 Sternal wires from cardiac surgery, with mitral valve replacement; now with heart failure, demonstrating Kerley B lines

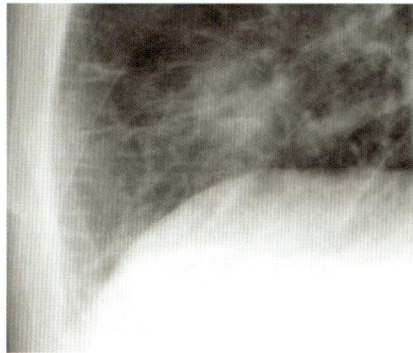

Figure 5.2 Kerley B lines as demonstrated on image above, magnified

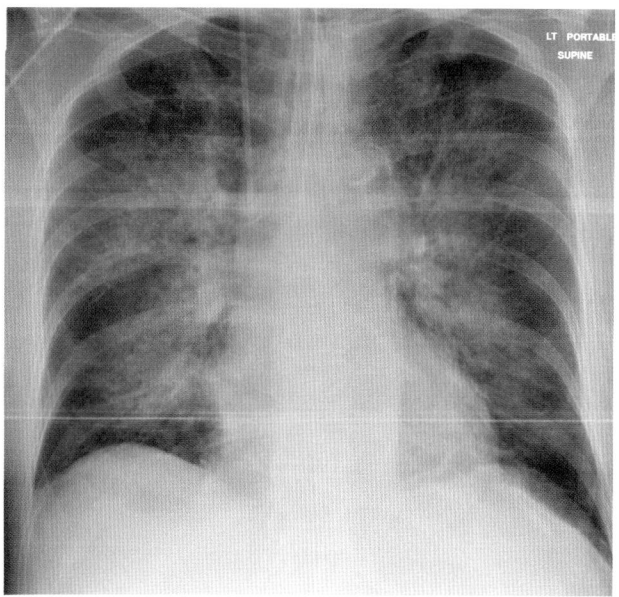

Figure 5.3 So-called 'bat wing' of pulmonary oedema

Valvular heart disease

Echocardiography is the image modality that enables the diagnosis.

Mitral stenosis and mitral incompetence

The chest x-ray may demonstrate left atrial enlargement, and sometimes calcification of the valve. The main use of the chest x-ray is to demonstrate raised pulmonary venous pressure and pulmonary oedema. Unless pulmonary hypertension develops, the transverse cardiac diameter is often normal. Pulmonary hypertension leads to other problems, such as dilation of the pulmonary arteries, and right ventricular enlargement. With mitral incompetence, the size of the left atrium corresponds well with the severity of the disease. The difference in chest x-ray appearance of mitral incompetence (compared with mitral stenosis) is the presence of left ventricular enlargement.

Aortic stenosis

The main features on the chest x-ray are aortic valve calcification and post-stenotic dilation of the ascending aorta. Left ventricular enlargement and raised pulmonary venous pressure are late signs, indicating left ventricular failure.

Aortic incompetence

Unlike aortic stenosis, aortic incompetence leads to enlargement of the left ventricle early in the disease. As the severity increases, the left atrium enlarges and raised pulmonary venous pressure develops.

Tricuspid stenosis and incompetence

Both these conditions result in enlargement of the right atrium and superior vena cava. They are rarely seen in isolation; there is often also mitral valve disease.

Left atrial myxoma

This is the commonest type of cardiac tumour, and is benign. It can interfere with the function of the mitral valve, thus mimicking mitral stenosis.

Ischaemic heart disease

Most patients with angina or myocardial infarction have a normal chest. The signs which may be present on a plain chest image are:
- Signs of raised pulmonary venous pressure and pulmonary oedema
- Cardiac enlargement, and aneurysm formation
- Myocardial infarcts occasionally calcify
- Atheromatous calcification may be seen in the coronary arteries.

Conclusion

This is an extensive and complicated subject and this chapter has only briefly reviewed some of the main cardiovascular disorders. It has mainly focused on some of the possible appearances of cardiac disease on the chest image, which enables identification of early cardiac disease.

Key points to remember

- *Remember how to measure CTR (see Chapter 1), its usefulness and limitations.*
- *Remember how to identify atrial enlargement, as well as pulmonary enlargement.*
- *Pulmonary venous hypertension is often caused by mitral valve disease, or LVF.*
- *Know how to identify pulmonary and interstitial oedema.*
- *Be able to identify Kerley A and B lines.*

LUNG TUMOURS

Introduction

This is a complex and lengthy subject so this chapter will only briefly review bronchogenic carcinoma. For further information, please refer to the many reference books on the subject (see p. 197 [References & Further Reading]). Risk factors for bronchogenic carcinoma are smoking, asbestos exposure and genetic predisposition. In the UK, according to Hunt *et al.* (2009) lung cancer among men has declined with the reduction in men smoking, but in women lung cancer rates continue to increase as proportionally more women smoke. Surprisingly, according to Hunt *et al.* (2009), more women die of lung cancer than breast cancer. Bronchogenic carcinoma is a generic term for several types of cancer, including adenocarcinoma, squamous cell carcinoma, small cell carcinoma and large cell carcinoma. Hunt *et al.* (2009) and De Lacey *et al.* (2008) provide useful tables regarding the frequency and location of these tumours. Some of this information (combined with information from other texts) has been used to formulate Table 6.1 below.

Table 6.1 Location and frequency of lung tumours

Type of tumour	Location	Further information
Adenocarcinoma	Peripheral	Scar carcinoma
Squamous cell carcinoma	Central, peripheral	Cavitations
Small cell carcinoma	Central, peripheral	Endocrine activity
Large cell carcinoma	Central, peripheral	Large mass

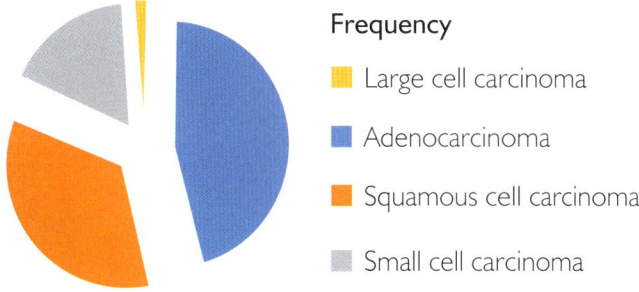

Figure 6.1 Frequency of lung tumours

This chapter will comment on some of the clinical signs of lung cancer, briefly review its diagnosis and staging, and discuss screening for lung cancer.

Some common clinical manifestations of lung cancer

Often the patient will first visit their General Practitioner (GP) with a cough lasting for more than 3 weeks; alternatively, the patient may have a cough that is not clearing, following treatment with antibiotics. This will lead to an initial chest x-ray being undertaken. Other clinical signs of a primary tumour are dyspnoea, chest discomfort and haemoptysis. Oesophageal symptoms or Horner's syndrome (drooping of the eyelid and constriction of the pupil, due to involvement of the sympathetic nerve) may be signs of intrathoracic spread of the primary lung tumour.

Clinical signs of Pancoast's tumour

This is a tumour located in the lung apex that has extended into the chest wall. Pancoast's tumours are often squamous cell carcinoma. Clinical signs include phrenic nerve paralysis, Horner's syndrome, recurrent laryngeal nerve paralysis (altered voice), pain radiating down the arm, and invasion of pleura, bone and brachial plexus or subclavian vessels.

Clinical signs of extrathoracic spread of lung cancer

The patient may experience a variety of symptoms, ranging from bone pain and fracture to confusion and personality change. There may also be focal neurological deficits, headaches, nausea, vomiting, palpable lymphadenopathy, seizure weakness and weight loss.

Chest x-ray features of lung tumours

Most nodules greater than 1cm will be defined on a chest x-ray; others may cause collapse, consolidation or a unilateral pleural effusion. The majority of bronchogenic carcinomas arise in larger bronchi at, or close to, the hilum; the remainder arise peripherally.

Signs of a central tumour

The tumour may present as a hilar mass, and/or narrowing of the main bronchus. The narrowing may be irregular or smooth; an irregular stricture is virtually diagnostic of a carcinoma. The effect of obstruction of a tumour is usually a combination of collapse and consolidation. The alveoli collapse because air is absorbed beyond the obstructed bronchus and cannot be replaced; consolidation is the result of retained secretions and secondary infection. If a chest x-ray demonstrates a patch of consolidation that does not clear with treatment, or a unilateral pleural effusion with no obvious underlying cause, you should therefore be highly suspicious of an underlying lung tumour, which may be hidden by the effusion or too small to be radiographically identified.

Signs of a peripheral tumour

This usually presents as a solitary pulmonary mass. A round shadow with an irregular border (lobulated, notching or infiltrating) is a common pattern for a bronchial carcinoma. Sometimes cavitations will occur within the mass; this tends to occur with peripheral squamous cell carcinomas. Typically, the walls of the cavity are thick and irregular.

Rapid increase in size

A doubling of volume in less than 3 months is unlikely to be a neoplasm, and much more likely to be an infective or inflammatory process. However, if the doubling time is from 3 to 18 months the lesion is more likely to be malignant (Ellis & Flower 2006).

De Lacey et al. (2008) correctly state that tumours will often hide and are overlapped by normal structures. Bearing this and the above information in mind, once the chest x-ray has been viewed, it is worth looking again even more carefully at the four areas De Lacey et al. (2008) comment on. These include the lung apices, looking especially for a Pancoast's tumour. The tumour may be overlapped by ribs, and a flat apical carcinoma can mimic a pleural cap; a pleural cap should not be deeper than 5mm, and both pleural caps should be about the same depth. You should look also carefully at adjacent ribs for tumour erosion. Other areas to review again, when looking for tumours, are behind the heart, below the diaphragm on the frontal radiograph (as a large proportion of the lower lobes of the lung lie below the horizon of the diaphragm), and of course around the hila.

Signs of spread of bronchial carcinoma

Hilar and mediastinal lymph node enlargement may occur, due to lymphatic spread of the tumour. Enlarged lymph nodes can be most readily identified at the hilum and the right paratracheal area. Although the lymph nodes would have to be extremely large to be identified on a chest x-ray, they can be identified on high-resolution computed tomography (HRCT). Pleural effusion may be due to malignant involvement of the pleura (or if on the opposite lung field to the primary tumour) may indicate malignant spread.

Invasion of the mediastinum may be indicated on the chest x-ray by widening of the mediastinal shadow and elevation of the hemidiaphragm due to phrenic nerve involvement. Invasion of the chest wall, may be demonstrated by destruction of an adjacent rib. The primary lung tumour may continue to metastasise to the ribs and/or other parts of the lung. Lymphangitis carcinomatosa is caused by blockage of the pulmonary lymphatics by carcinomatous tissue. The lymphatic vessels become grossly distended and the lungs become oedematous, but the heart remains its normal size and there is hilar adenopathy and/or lobar consolidation.

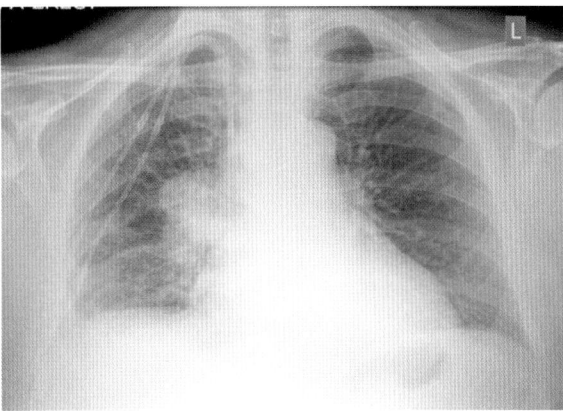

Figure 6.2 Right hilar tumour with lymphangitis

Lung cancer investigations

Once the chest x-ray has raised the suspicion of a bronchogenic carcinoma, the patient will be put onto a lung cancer fast-track programme and a HRCT scan will be performed. This will provide more information regarding the suspected bronchogenic carcinoma, such as:

- Determining whether it is malignant
- If so, determining whether it has spread
- It will also allow staging of the carcinoma.

In order to obtain further information regarding the type and spread of the tumour prior to treatment, other investigations may be required. These may include a bronchoscopy, a biopsy and sometimes a positron emission tomography (PET) scan. As it becomes more readily available, PET scanning is frequently used to evaluate indeterminate lung nodules, allowing differentiation between benign or malignant. PET scanning uses the radionuclide fluorine 18 fluorodeoxyglucose (PDG), which is introduced into the patient who is then scanned. This radionuclide is preferentially taken up and trapped in metabolically active cells, such as malignant tumours. Imaging is then done with a PET scanner.

The PET scanner can evaluate nodules as small as 8mm in diameter. The sensitivity of these PET scanners, and the use of PDG in detecting malignancy, is 95% successful for nodules 1cm or larger. However, its specificity is lower, as other metabolic cells (such as those found in infections) can also take up the PDG. Once all these investigations are done, the case will be discussed at a lung multidisciplinary team meeting to decide on a treatment pathway. The radiologists involved will need to stage the tumour for the clinical team.

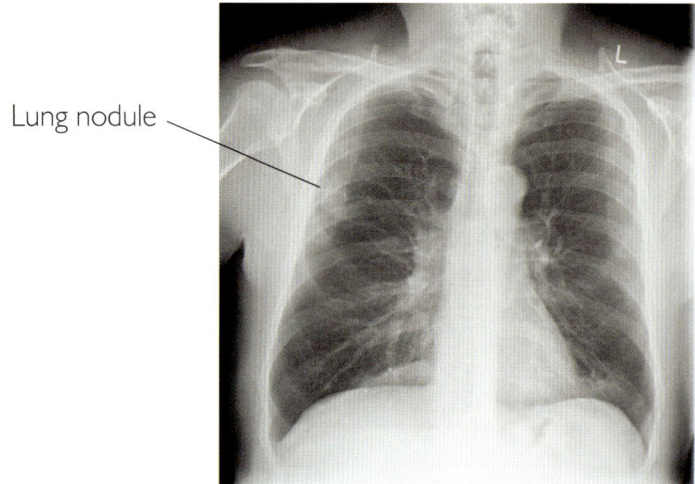

Figure 6.3 Chest x-ray following a cough for several weeks; right upper zone opacity demonstrated; this may be consolidation or a lung nodule

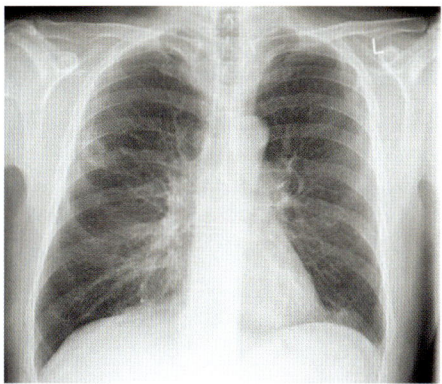

Figure 6.4 Repeat chest x-ray 4 weeks later; nodule appears to be cavitating – most likely lung cancer

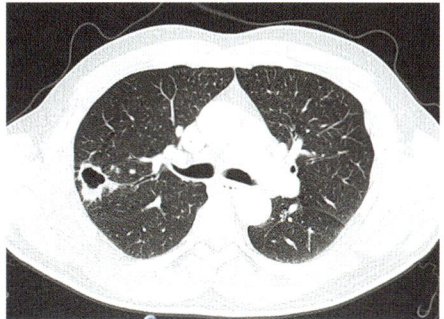

Figure 6.5 HRCT followed, demonstrating T2a N0 M0 lung cancer

Summary of the TNM staging system

There is a set way of staging the diagnosed lung tumour, which identifies the size of the tumour, its extension into surrounding areas, and whether there is lymph node involvement or metastases. This tells the clinician whether or not the tumour is resectable and indicates the 5-year survival rate. Many textbooks document this staging system. It is too lengthy to discuss in detail here but a quick summary appears below. **T** stands for the primary lung tumour, **N** indicates lymph node involvement and **M** refers to whether or not metastases are present.

Primary tumour (T):
- T0 – no evidence of primary tumour
- T1 – less than 3cm, limited to lung
- T2 – between 3 and 7 cm
- T3 – tumour of any size, with direct invasion to:
  - Chest wall, superior sulcus, diaphragm
  - Pleura, pericardium
  - Within 2cm of carina
- T4 – mediastinal organs, carinal, vertebral body invasion or malignant pleural effusion.

Nodes:
- N0 – no lymph node involvement
- N1 – ipsilateral peri bronchial or hilar nodes
- N2 – ipsilateral mediastinal or subcarinal nodes
- N3 – contra lateral hilar or mediastinal nodes; subclavicular nodes.

Metastases:
- M0 – no metastases
- M1 – distant metastases
- M1a – metastases in contralateral lobe
- M1b – distant metastases.

Unresectable stages:
- Tumours are unresectable if T4, N3 or M1
- Stage 3b – N3, M0, any T, T4, M0, any T
- Stage 4 – M1, any T, any N.

5-year survival:
- Stage 1 – 60%
- Stage 2 – 40%
- Stage 3a (limited disease) – 20%
- Stage 3b, 4 – 0%

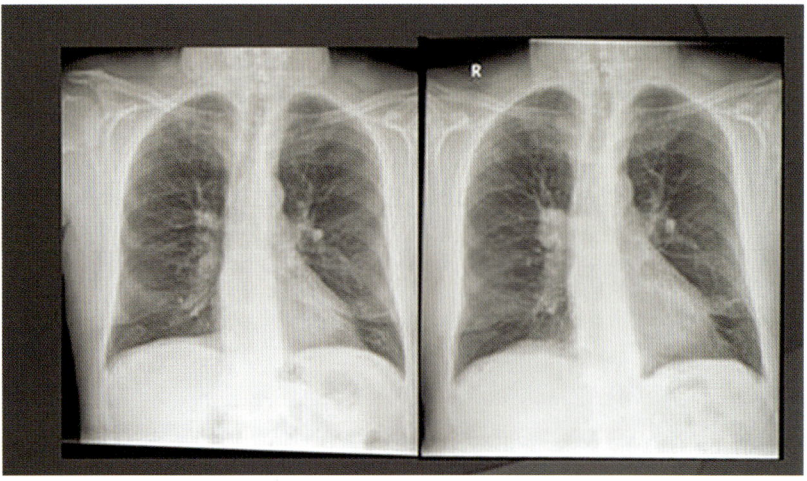

Original x-ray   6 week follow-up

Figure 6.6 Chest x-ray demonstrated subtle right upper zone consolidation; repeat x-ray after 6 weeks demonstrated enlarged right hilar and consolidation reduced; this case demonstrates the importance of reviewing all old images

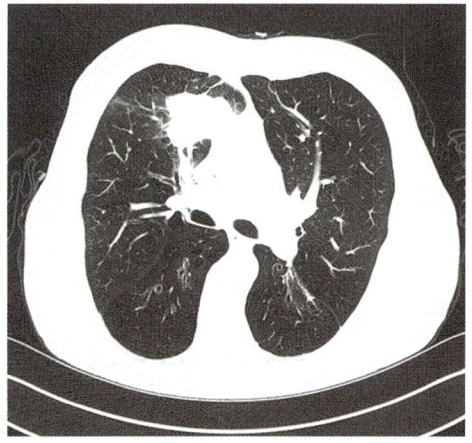

Figure 6.7 HRCT followed

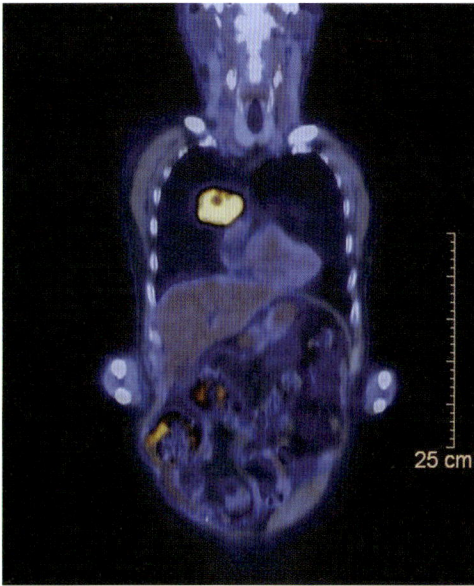

Figure 6.8 The HRCT was followed by a PET and a lung biopsy; T2b N0 M0

Screening programmes

In the Leeds Trust, a research programme into lung tumour screening was started in 2010. Patients are able to self-refer for a chest x-ray if they meet certain criteria: over 50 years of age; not having had a chest x-ray in the last 3 months; and having had a cough (or any of the other listed symptoms) for more than 3 weeks. The other symptoms include breathlessness, change in voice, coughing up blood, loss of weight and chest pain, which are all symptoms of lung cancer, but also of other conditions. The self-referral form is checked by the radiographer to ensure it fits the criteria before the chest x-ray is done. Whether or not the patient smokes is also documented.

This research was originally started because lung cancer is often picked up earlier in Europe than in the UK. The earlier it is diagnosed, the better the prognosis; and the research aims to address this. The NICE guidelines (2005) had already suggested when an urgent chest x-ray should be requested:

- Cough
- Chest/shoulder pain
- Dyspnoea
- Weight loss
- Hoarseness
- Finger clubbing
- Chest signs
- Cervical/supraclavicular lymphadenopathy
- Features suggestive of metastatic disease
- Haemoptysis.

The government had set guidelines for secondary care – 62 days from referral to start of treatment. However, the delay seemed to occur in primary care and patient delay in attending. Research was done into reasons for patient delay in attending, and the two main reasons given were 'difficulty making an appointment with GP' and 'did not want to waste doctor's time' – hence the start of the self-referral chest x-ray.

The centres running the programmes were set up in so-called deprived areas, where it was felt that patients might not normally attend the GP's surgery with signs of lung cancer. These areas were also thought to have a high incidence of smoking. The self-referral chest x-ray service was widely advertised, and many patients presented for chest x-rays. Some lung cancers were picked up but not the percentage expected. The self-referral service continues but it is no longer a government-funded research project. However, other Trusts in the UK have shown interest in the self-referral chest x-ray scheme. Further research is being done into the use of CT in screening for lung cancer.

Lung tumour screening programmes are constantly debated; interestingly Manser and his colleagues (2009) commented in their conclusion that they did not support screening for lung cancer, and that too many chest x-rays might be detrimental. However, these days the dose of a chest x-ray with digital equipment has been reduced to such an extent that you are likely to receive more radiation dose from a single flight to Spain than from a chest x-ray. The level of detail in these digital images has also been greatly increased.

Ketai *et al.* (2006) disagree with lung cancer screening with CT, as the dose is much higher than that from a chest x-ray. However, their main reason for disagreeing with lung cancer screening with CT is not the radiation dose but the fact that CT demonstrates so many small nodules. These result in being followed up with serial CT scans over a 2-year period and then turn out to be benign and the process becomes unmanageable. The high rate of false positives led to Ketai *et al.* (2006) concluding that CT screening should not be done for lung tumours, especially in low-risk patients. Edey and Hansell (2009) also found that CT detects lots of incidental small pulmonary nodules.

More recent lung cancer CT screening trials in US and Europe, using low-dose CT in high-risk individuals, have seen significant reduction in lung cancer. The European trial (Zhao 2011) demonstrated a 26% mortality reduction in high-risk men and 61% in high-risk women. The Yorkshire lung screening trial has now opened to screen 7,000 high-risk patients.

Conclusion

Further research into the use of low-dose CT in certain high-risk patients is currently being carried out. Nelson's study of lung cancer screening CT in high-risk individuals has already shown positive results (Zhao 2011). It will be interesting to see how these results compare with those of the Yorkshire trial in the future. However, it does seem clear that the earlier lung cancer is diagnosed, the better the prognosis. Whoever is reviewing the chest x-ray (whatever the clinical request is) should always make a thorough search for any evidence of a lung tumour. Any slight suspicions of lung cancer on the chest x-ray should be followed up rapidly with a HRCT scan; and the patient should be put on a lung cancer fast-track programme, to ensure the best outcome.

Key points to remember:

- *Know the clinical signs of lung cancer.*
- *Know possible chest x-ray features of lung cancer.*
- *A doubling of volume in less than 3 months is unlikely to be a neoplasm, and much more likely to be an infective or inflammatory process. However, if the doubling time is from 3 to 18 months the lesion is more likely to be malignant (Ellis & Flower 2006).*
- *Look for signs of spread of lung cancer.*
- *Know your local protocols for alerting for lung cancer.*
- *Be aware of staging for lung cancer.*

IF IN DOUBT, ASK.

LUNG NODULES

Introduction

Around 80% of solitary lung nodules are granuloma or bronchial cancer (Ketai et al. 2006). Lung tumours have already been discussed in the previous chapter, so they will not be further discussed here. We shall now briefly review some of the other (mainly benign) causes of a solitary lung nodule. For more in-depth information, please refer to the many reference texts on this subject.

Other causes of a solitary lung nodule are bronchial carcinoids, hamartomas, round atelectasis, organising pneumonia and pulmonary infarct. This chapter will mainly use a selection of texts to briefly describe each of the causes of a solitary lung nodule. This, along with the previous chapter on lung tumours, will help in differentiating the many causes of a solitary lung nodule, as well as being helpful in ascertaining whether a particular lung nodule has a benign or malignant cause.

Ketai et al. (2006) provide an excellent table of the common causes of solitary pulmonary nodules which is summarised below, along with information from other texts (De Lacey et al. 2008, Weissleder 1997).

Table 7.1 Common causes of solitary pulmonary nodules (excluding bronchial cancer)

Diagnosis	Radiological clues to diagnosis
Most common	
Granuloma	Dense central calcifications occupying more than 20% of nodule
Sarcoid granuloma	Look for other signs of sarcoid, such as enlarged hilar
Wegener's granuloma	More common in middle to lower lung
Less common	
Solitary metastases	Endobronchial location, marked enhancement after intravenous contrast.
Bronchial carcinoid	
Hamartoma	Intra-lesion fat on CT
Rounded atelectasis	Must be adjacent to pleural thickening
Organising pneumonia	May have concave borders

De Lacey et al. (2008) expand on Ketai et al.'s (2006) possible causes of a solitary pulmonary nodule by including some other less common causes, such as abscess, infected bullae, infarct, rheumatoid nodule; and then some very rare causes, such as arterio-venous malformation, intrapulmonary lipoma, amyloid and hydatid cyst.

Granulomas

Often the frequency of granulomas and bronchogenic carcinoma depends on the age of the patient and their smoking history. Granulomas have a classic radiographic appearance with a calcified central nidus; unfortunately, some may remain uncalcified; Ketai et al. (2006) comment that this occurs more commonly with coccidiomycosis, than other fungi or mycobacteria. Plasma cell granuloma, according to Weissleder et al. (1997), is a local cellular proliferation of spindle cells, plasma cells, lymphocytes and histiocytes in the lung. It is the most common tumour-like pulmonary abnormality in children less than 15 years of age and has very slow growth or no growth.

Wegener's granulomatosis, although included in De Lacey et al.'s (2008) differential of a solitary pulmonary nodule, normally presents with multiple nodules with cavitations. It initially appears as interstitial, reticulonodular opacities at the lung bases. Sarcoid granuloma, again in De Lacey et al.'s (2008) differential, is more likely to produce multiple granuloma, often in the mid and upper zones, and has associated hilar and paratracheal lymphadenopathy.

Hamartomas

Hamartomas are benign tumours, mainly composed of cartilage, connective tissue, muscle, fat and bone. According to Weissleder et al. (1997), 90% are peripheral and 10% are endobronchial. Hamartomas are normally well-circumscribed, solitary nodules, with classically popcorn calcification, but this occurs in less than 20% of cases. However, fat attenuation within a lesion is pathognomonic (demonstrated on CT). They are the most common benign non-inflammatory cause of a solitary pulmonary nodule (Ketai et al. 2006). They most commonly occur in patients aged 45 to 50 years of age, and constitute 5% of resected nodules (Ketai et al. 2006).

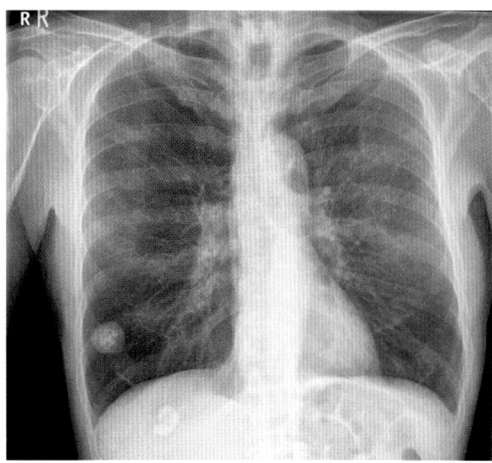

Figure 7.1 Classic appearance of hamartoma with popcorn calcification in right lower zone

Bronchial carcinoid

Bronchial carcinoid is not a benign lesion, but a low-grade malignancy, representing 90% of low-grade tumours of the lungs. The 10-year survival rate with surgical treatment is 85% (Weissleder et al. 1997). There are two types: Type I is typical carcinoid and remains a local tumour; Type II, atypical carcinoid (10–20%), metastasises to regional lymph nodes, but liver metastases are very rare.

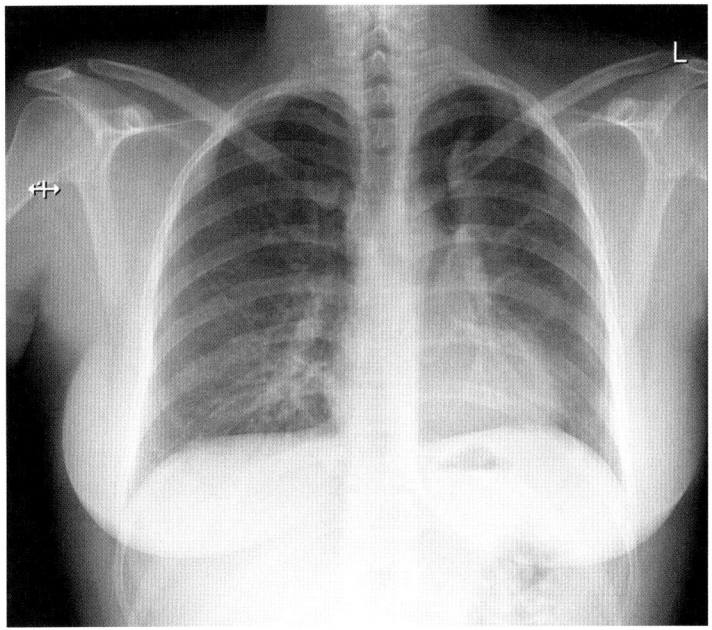

Figure 7.2 Chest x-ray for breathlessness and cough. Demonstrates left upper lobe collapse, with classic 'veil-like appearance', and loss of clearly defined left heart border. Collapse of the lung can be a result of many causes, such as mucous plug, lung nodule, etc.

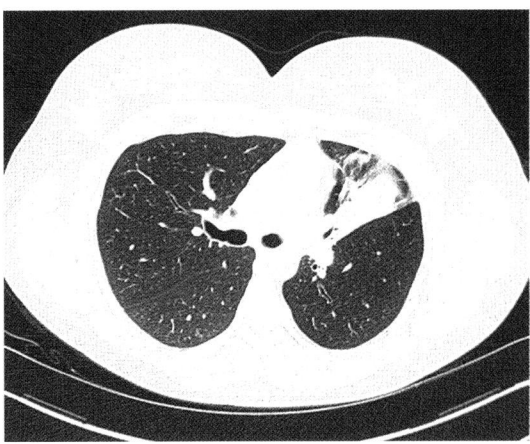

Figure 7.3 High-resolution computed tomography (HRCT) followed, demonstrating a carcinoid

Solitary metastasis

Suspicion arises that the solitary pulmonary nodule is a solitary metastasis if there is a known extra-thoracic malignancy. The most common malignancy to present as a solitary lung metastasis is from colon carcinoma. It is important to determine whether the lung nodule is a lung metastasis or a primary lung carcinoma (see Chapter 6). In general, a previous squamous cell carcinoma of the head and neck is more likely to result in a new bronchogenic carcinoma than a metastasis. However, in patients with previous colon or renal carcinoma, a solitary metastasis and a new bronchogenic occur equally commonly. Patients with soft tissue sarcomas or melanomas are more likely to have a solitary metastasis than a primary lung tumour. It is possible that a primary lung carcinoma can also metastasise, sometimes to the opposite lung.

Rounded atelectasis

These often occur in patients with asbestos-related pleural disease. This diagnosis should be considered when the pulmonary nodule lies next to an area of pleural thickening. According to Ketai et al. (2006), this type of atelectasis occurs when a section of the lung parenchyma becomes engulfed by the pleura, often during resolution of a pleural effusion (as always, previous images are helpful in this case). However, on occasions, it can occur in non-asbestos-related pleural disease.

Pneumonia

Acute pneumonia is a rare cause of pulmonary nodule, but may occur in an immune-compromised adult following infection with an atypical organism, such as Aspergillus. A round pneumonia may be seen in paediatrics, often secondary to pneumococcus.

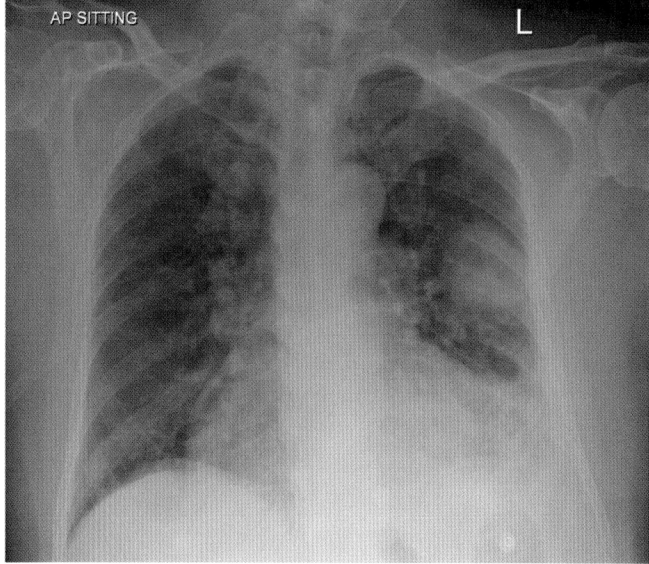

Figure 7.4 Patient with advanced pneumonia in both lungs and left basal effusion; also demonstrated at the left mid zone is rounded consolidation/pneumonia

Pulmonary infarct

A pulmonary infarct caused by an embolus may cause a solitary lung nodule, but this is a rare cause. More often, an infarct produces multiple opacities. De Lacey *et al.* (2008) comment on 'traps' that may simulate pulmonary nodules. Below is their definitive list. Most of these are obviously *not* a solitary pulmonary nodule, but some can be relatively easily mistaken for one, so they are included here for the sake of completeness.

Things that may simulate pulmonary nodules on a chest x-ray:

- Overlap of normal pulmonary vessels
- Healing rib fracture
- Rib density – benign
- Rib density – malignant
- Pleural plaque
- Encysted pleural fluid
- Electrocardiogram electrode pad
- Nipple shadow
- Skin mole
- Clothing artefact.

Conclusion

This chapter has briefly outlined some of the causes of a solitary lung nodule, apart from bronchial carcinoma. Often a chest x-ray alone is not enough to arrive at a definite diagnosis. A list of differentials, CT, PET scans and sometimes biopsy may also be required. This chapter (together with Chapter 6 on lung tumours) helps in identifying a lung nodule and writing a differential diagnosis, as well as suggesting further imaging in order to provide a definitive diagnosis on a solitary lung nodule.

Key points to remember

- *Around 80% of solitary lung nodules are granuloma or bronchial carcinoma.*
- *Other causes of a solitary lung nodule are bronchial carcinoid, hamartomas, rounded atelectasis, organising pulmonary pneumonia, pleural infarct.*
- *Be aware of appearance of a solitary metastasis.*
- *Be aware of things that may simulate the appearance of a lung nodule, e.g. pleural plaque, rib fracture or anomaly, nipple shadow, etc.*

CHEST TRAUMA

Introduction

This chapter will mainly concentrate on blunt trauma of the chest, following major trauma. The most common major trauma is a road traffic collision (RTC). RTCs are the third most common cause of death worldwide, causing more than 1 million deaths and 38 million injuries each year. They can occur in many ways – vehicle versus vehicle, vehicle versus pedestrian, vehicle versus stationary object, and motorcycle and cycle injuries.

It is important for the A&E clinician to obtain an accurate assessment of the incident scene in order to predict a pattern of injuries. They need to know (Brooks, Mahoney & Hodgetts 2007):

- The estimated speed of impact
- The type of collision, i.e. frontal, side or rear
- Position of patient within vehicle, i.e. driver, or front or rear seat passenger
- Did the vehicle roll over?
- Were the occupants wearing seatbelts?
- Were they ejected? If so, how far?
- Did the car have airbags that were deployed?
- How long did it take to get the injured people out of the car?
- The type of vehicle and the extent of damage to it.

Injury to the chest is common in an RTC; in fact, in a high-speed road traffic collision, aortic rupture is the most common cause of sudden death. The descending aorta is relatively fixed in position but the aortic arch is unsupported. Therefore, a sudden deceleration can cause the aortic arch to shear off from the descending aorta, resulting in an injury which is usually fatal within seconds (Greaves, Porter & Ryan 2001).

At this stage, it is important to remember the basic laws of motion and the types of fractures that are most likely to occur.

The basic laws of motion

Injuries occur as a result of the transfer of **kinetic energy** (KE), which is the energy of motion. This can be defined as: **KE** $= \frac{1}{2}mv^2$ where **m = mass** and **v = velocity.**

This and the information obtained from the trauma scene, be it an RTC or a fall from a height, etc. allows the clinician to predict not only the range of injuries but their likely severity.

De Lacey *et al.* (2008) comment that there are eight main things to look for:
- Fractures
- Pneumothorax
- Pneumomediastinum
- Aortic rupture
- Tracheo-bronchial injury
- Lung contusion
- Cardiac trauma
- Ruptured diaphragm.

These are the areas we shall be briefly reviewing in this chapter.

Fractures

Rib fractures occur in 10% of RTC patients and are associated with morbidity and mortality (Whitson *et al.* 2012). The first fractures to look for on the chest x-ray are fractured ribs. They may be associated with extra-pleural soft tissue swelling due to bruising, or frank haematoma may be present. Be careful not to mistake this appearance for a pleural mass.

Carefully review the first three ribs, remembering also the clavicle and scapula, as fractures in this area are indicative of a severe force. There are several soft tissues nearby which may also be injured (if the trauma is severe enough), namely the subclavian artery, bronchus and brachial plexus. If the lower ribs are fractured, they may lacerate the kidneys, spleen or liver.

The ribs should also be assessed for a flail segment (defined as two fractures in each of two or more adjacent ribs). A flail segment may sometimes not be radiographically visualised because one of the fractures is through rib cartilage or at the costochondral junction. The clinical importance of a flail segment is that it may cause paradoxical movement of the adjacent lung, which can adversely affect gas exchange (De Lacey *et al.* 2008, Ketai *et al.* 2006, Weissleder *et al.* 1997).

Whitson *et al.* (2012), when researching whether increasing numbers of rib fractures increase morbidity, concluded that the age of the patient and overall trauma burden were more powerful predictors of morbidity. They did not highlight in their research whether the site of the fractured rib had any influence on morbidity. For instance, as mentioned earlier, a fracture of the first rib may puncture the subclavian artery; whereas fractures of the lower ribs may injure the spleen, kidney or liver, thus increasing the likelihood of serious consequences. Perhaps this is an area for further research. Channey *et al.* (2012) investigated whether patients with rib fractures developed delayed pneumonia, and concluded that they did not.

A fractured rib can of course result in a pneumothorax, haemothorax or lung contusion, and these should be actively searched for on the chest radiograph.

The dorsal spine is included on the chest x-ray, so it is important to review it. The dorsal spine will probably need windowing to view adequately and you should also check the paraspinal line to look for fracture, as fracture of the dorsal spine is a major trauma.

Minor trauma may result in displaced/minimally displaced rib fractures which are of limited clinical significance, with the Royal College of Radiologists (2012) agreeing that in cases of minor trauma the demonstration of a simple rib fracture will not alter management, and a chest x-ray should not be done unless a pneumothorax or infection is suspected. Reuter (1996) noted that most fractures tend to be of the posterior or lateral 6th, 7th or 8th rib, which are normally well seen on a chest x-ray.

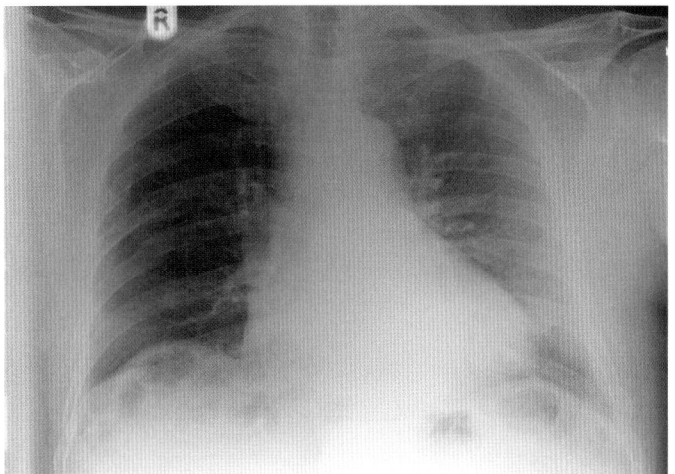

Figure 8.1 Multiple right-sided posterior rib fractures

Pneumothorax

Pneumothorax may occur if the lung is punctured by a direct injury or the edge of a fractured rib. Following major trauma, the patient will be x-rayed supine, and air collects at the highest point which will be anteriorly. The person reviewing the chest image needs to look carefully for the deep sulcus sign (i.e. the anterior costophrenic angle sharply delineated). It is important to detect even a small pneumothorax if the patient is to be treated with positive pressure ventilation, to prevent their small pneumothorax becoming a large one.

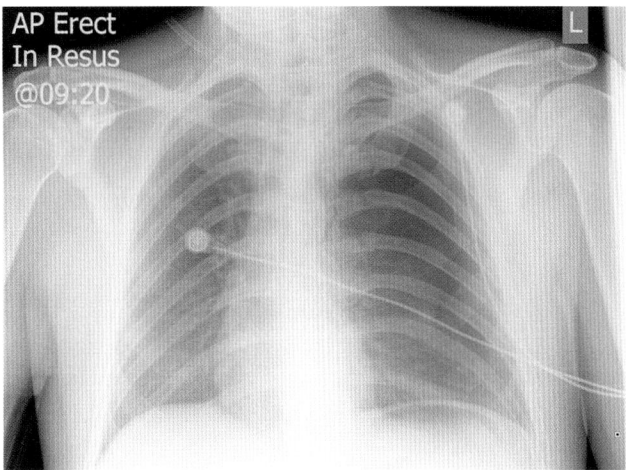

Figure 8.2 A large left-sided pneumothorax; patient x-rayed in a sitting position; the heart appears to be moving to the right side

The chest image should also be assessed for a tension pneumothorax. The radiographic features of a tension pneumothorax are over-expanded lung, depressed diaphragm and shift of the mediastinum and heart to the contra-lateral side. However, some say that you should never see a chest x-ray of a tension pneumothorax, as it should be treated clinically before x-ray.

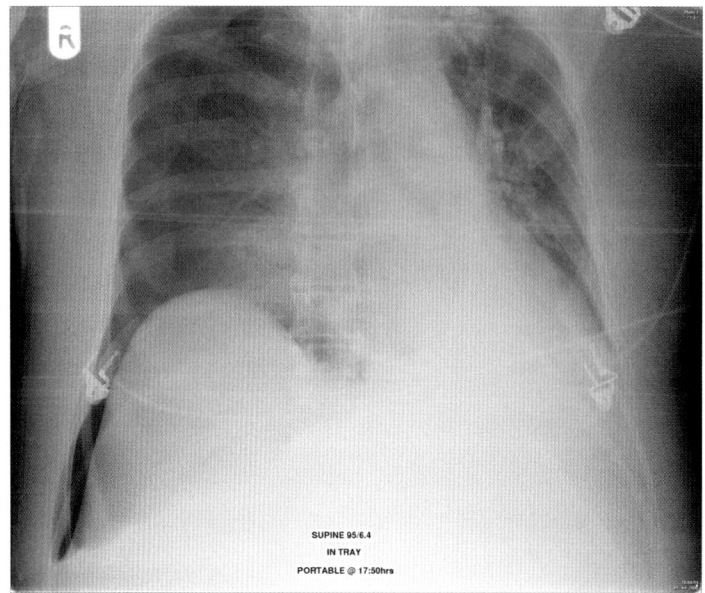

Figure 8.3 A large right-sided pneumothorax; patient x-rayed in a supine position, demonstrating the deep sulcus sign

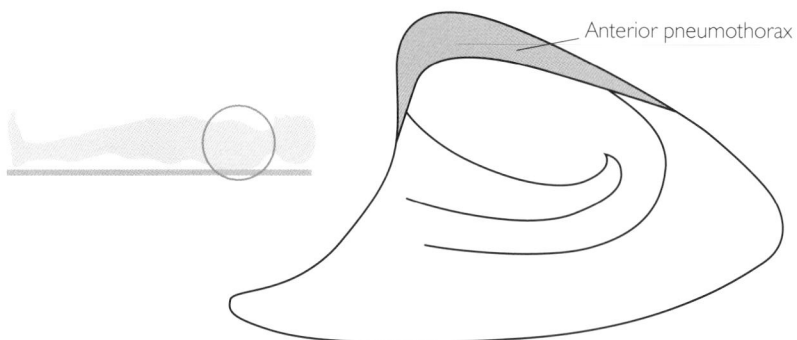

Figure 8.4 Anterior pneumothorax, lateral view. Remember, in a supine patient air rises

Pneumomediastinum

Pneumomediastinum can be recognised by displacement of the mediastinal pleura laterally, which creates a dark line next to the heart and mediastinal structures. Dark streaks of air are often seen extending upwards towards the neck; dark lines may also encircle the right pulmonary artery on the lateral view, causing a ring around the artery. The patient is likely to be supine when the chest x-ray is taken, so visualisation of the central portion of the diaphragm (the continuous diaphragm sign) can be a useful clue to the presence of a pneumomediastinum (De Lacey et al. 2008, Ketai et al. 2006, Weissleder et al. 1997).

In a major trauma situation, pneumomediastinum may result from a tear of the lung tissue, pneumothorax, rupture of trachea or bronchus, rupture of oesophagus, or rupture of the intra-abdominal viscus. If serial chest x-rays demonstrate a persistent severe pneumomediastinum, an unrecognised rupture of oesophagus or trachea-bronchial rupture should be suspected.

Aortic rupture

Around 80–90% of patients with an aortic rupture die immediately (De Lacey et al. 2008). Some appearances on the chest x-ray to look for that may suggest aortic rupture include:
- Widened mediastinum
- Trachea displaced to the right
- Lobulated aortic outline
- A haemothorax
- An apical pleural cap.

Tracheo-bronchial rupture

These ruptures are usually from a high-speed RTC, and are usually the result of a deceleration force applied to the chest wall. You should also look for associated fractures of the sternum and anterior ribs. These patients have a high mortality rate. The injury may result in a broncho-pleural fistula, and eventually bronchostenosis.

Features to look for on the chest x-ray include (De Lacey et al. 2008, Ketai et al. 2006, Weissleder et al. 1997):
- Pneumomediastinum
- Lobar collapse, which may not occur for a few days
- Pneumothorax that does not resolve.

Lung contusion

Lung contusion is due to endothelial damage causing blood to enter the interstitium and alveoli. It is mainly located next to solid structures, e.g. the ribs, heart and vertebrae. It occurs about 6–24 hours after the initial injury, and normally resolves 7–10 days later. The appearance on the radiograph is normally that of consolidation, which may cavitate. The appearance of consolidation may of course have other causes, such as adult respiratory distress syndrome (ARDS), fat emboli (which often follow chest trauma) or aspiration pneumonia (De Lacey et al. 2008, Ketai et al. 2006, Weissleder et al. 1997).

A patient with a lung contusion may sometimes later develop ARDS. Becher and his colleagues (2012) used software to measure the size of a lung contusion in a trauma patient to predict the likely development of ARDS. They discovered that patients with 24% or greater lung contusions were more likely to develop ARDS.

Cardiac trauma

The sternum, dorsal spine and pericardium protect the heart, so if there are fractures in these areas, there may be cardiac trauma. A pneumopericardium should also be searched for on the chest x-ray. With this condition, air surrounds the heart but does not extend upwards past the great vessels (unlike a pneumomediastinum). Echocardiography is more useful than a chest x-ray when looking for myocardial injury.

Rupture of the diaphragm

This occurs in 5% of cases of severe trauma. A rupture of the diaphragm may affect either dome but the left is more commonly affected. Some radiographic features to look for include:

- Air fluid levels above the diaphragm
- Abnormal elevation of the left hemidiaphragm (check against previous images)
- Abnormal contour of dome of diaphragm
- Centrolateral tension displacement of mediastinum
- Abnormal location of a nasogastric tube.

Several texts suggest arranging a coronal MRI to confirm the rupture of the diaphragm. In about 50% of cases, herniation of abdominal viscera through the rupture is delayed, sometimes by years (De Lacey *et al.* 2008, Ketai *et al.* 2006, Weissleder *et al.* 1997).

Conclusion

This has only been a brief review of the areas and types of injuries to look for on a post-traumatic chest x-ray. Today there are trauma centres throughout the UK, where patients from major RTCs are taken. Often at these sites if the trauma to the patient is significant, a trauma CT will be carried out in preference to plain films. However, chest x-rays are still carried out on some trauma patients, as they are quick and readily available. This chapter has concentrated on the basics of reviewing a chest image for evidence of the different types of chest trauma. However, it is still vital that the reviewer of the chest image is skilled in recognising these at an early stage in the treatment process, to ensure a good patient outcome.

Key points to remember

- *Know the 8 main things to look for in a trauma patient.*
- *When assessing fractured ribs, look for a flail segment.*
- *Remember, when looking for a pneumothorax, it will look different depending on the position of the patient.*
- *Also check for a haemothorax/effusion at the site of any fracture.*
- *Know what to look for in aortic rupture/ tracheo-bronchial rupture/diaphragmatic rupture.*
- *In severe trauma, the patient will often have a trauma CT scan.*

TUBES, LINES AND PACEMAKERS

Introduction

Evaluation of the placement of various tubes, wires and lines is a common reason for taking a chest x-ray. Often the image can look confusing with wires all over the place. However, it is imperative that the reader of the image assesses whether all the lines are in the right place. A misplaced line can lead to various significant complications, ranging from cardiac arrhythmias to lobar collapse. Often, these patients are very ill and in the intensive care unit (ICU). The chest image that is being reviewed will be anterior posterior, probably supine, and may be somewhat rotated, making assessment difficult.

This chapter brings together information obtained from texts, articles, lectures, chest radiologists and anaesthetists on intensive care and essentially documents the correct position for the various lines, and the complications that can result from misplaced lines.

Endotracheal (ET) tube

This is probably the easiest tube to identify, as it should be in the air shadow of the trachea. In an adult or child, the ET tip should be at least 1cm above the carina (Mettler 1996); and in an adult preferably 5–7cm (De Lacey et al. 2008) above the carina. An ET tube in a low position will usually go into the right bronchus, resulting in lung collapse. The highest that an ET tube tip should be is at the level of the suprasternal notch, midway between the proximal clavicles.

However, the ET tube can move up or down, depending on the position of the neck. In an adult, if you flex the neck, the tip can move 1.9cm downwards; extend the neck and it can move 1.9cm upwards; rotate the neck and it can move 0.7cm upwards (De Lacey et al. 2008). When taking a chest x-ray of an adult on the ICU in our Trust, the head is left in situ and nothing is documented about what position the head is in, although one can often work it out from the radiograph. Ideally the chest x-ray should be taken with the patient's head straight, so the ET tube is demonstrated in its correct position. However, it is obviously not ideal to ask the nurse to move an intensive care patient's head; so the radiographer should perhaps document on the chest x-ray image the position of the patient's head to help the reader/reporter of the image.

Interestingly on Paediatric ICU, the patient's head is placed centrally for the chest x-ray. This is an area for further research. Does moving the patient's head more result in the ET inadvertently moving, leading to it being in the wrong place? Or, as there is a relatively wide variant of normal ET tube placement in an adult, does it matter where the head is placed for the radiograph? Movement of the head in a neonate can result in the ET tube moving upwards by 1cm and hence being pulled out (Mettler 1996, Steiner 1993a).

Nasogastric (NG) tube

Nasogastric tubes are used for feeding the patient and for gastric decompression/aspiration. The NG tube should follow the course of the oesophagus and the tip should be positioned at least 5cm beyond the oesophago-gastric junction, in order to ensure that the side holes of the tube are not situated in the intra-abdominal part of the oesophagus.

Sometimes the NG tube may be curled up on itself, not far enough in or too far in; or (in the worst-case scenario) in the trachea and bronchus, resulting in lobar collapse; or if feeding through the tube without checking, aspiration pneumonia and probably lung collapse as well. It is therefore vital to check the position of the NG tube.

As a 2011 NHS safety alert commented, a misplaced nasogastric tube in an adult or child can result not only in significant harm but death (NHS NPSA 2011). The paper sets out action for the NHS to reduce the harm caused by misplaced nasogastric tubes, mainly commenting on a need for staff training and competency frameworks, not only regarding the insertion of the tube but also in the reviewing of the radiograph to ensure it is correctly placed, prior to feeding. The article also comments that all nasogastric tubes should be radio-opaque. This highlights the importance of radiographer practitioners and/or radiographers being trained in recognising the correct placement of nasogastric tubes, as it will enable them to make an important contribution to patient care and safety.

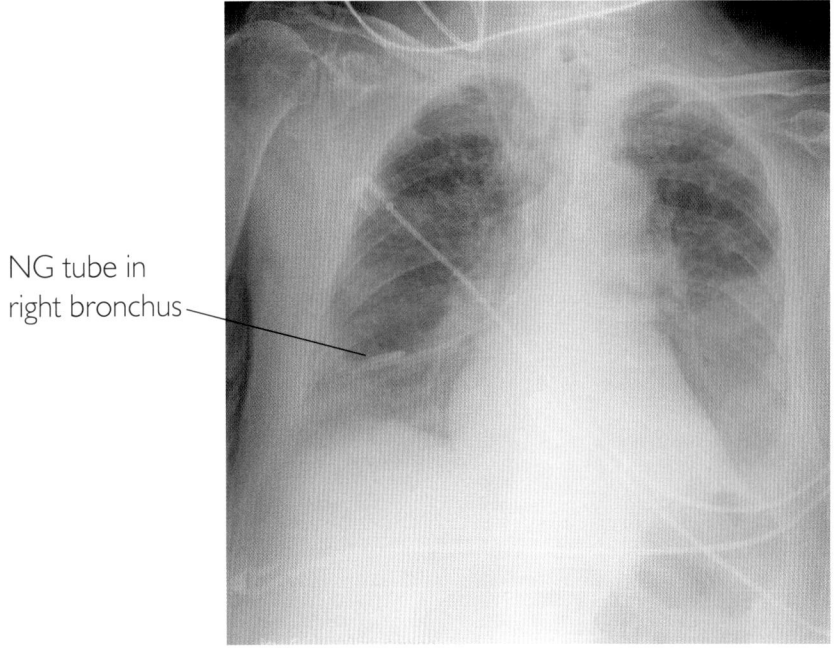

Figure 9.1 NG tube in right bronchus intermedius and beyond

At the Leeds Trust, several initiatives have been taken to prevent the above happening. Firstly, at the two main hospital sites, radiographers are trained to comment on the correct position of an NG tube on the chest x-ray that they have taken and document this information on the computer. If two radiographers decide that the NG tube is in an unsafe position, it is removed by the radiographers. Please see the following protocol regarding information entered by the radiographer commenting on the NG tube.

Following is the information taught to radiographers commenting on NG tubes, summarised in questions on four chest x-rays.

RADIOGRAPHER COMMENT ON NASOGASTRIC TUBE POSITION

THIS IS NOT A REPORT ON THE LUNGS AND MEDIASTINUM - A FORMAL RADIOLOGY REPORT CAN BE OBTAINED ON REQUEST

Aspirate details: UNABLE TO ASPIRATE / pH 6 OR MORE / OTHER

The tube follows the line of the oesophagus: YES / NO
The tube bisects the carina: YES / NO
The tip passes at least 5cm below the diaphragm: YES / NO
The crossing point is in the midline: YES / NO

LTHT GUIDELINES STATE THAT THE TUBE IS IN A SAFE POSITION TO FEED IF THE ANSWER TO ALL FOUR QUESTIONS IS YES

THE DECISION TO FEED LIES WITH WARD STAFF.

Has the ward been contacted: YES / NO
Name of ward staff contacted (if applicable):
Name of radiographer completing auto report:
Name of second person making decision to remove tube (if applicable):

Additional comments:

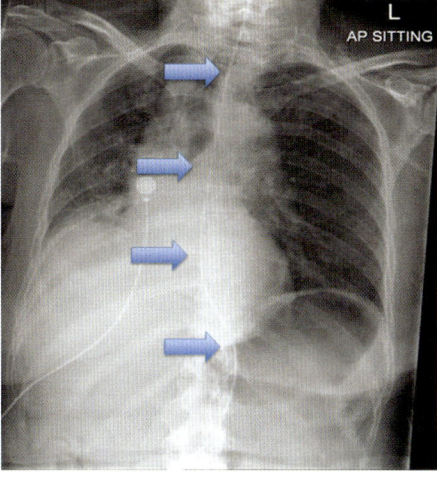

Figure 9.2 Does it follow the path of the oesophagus?

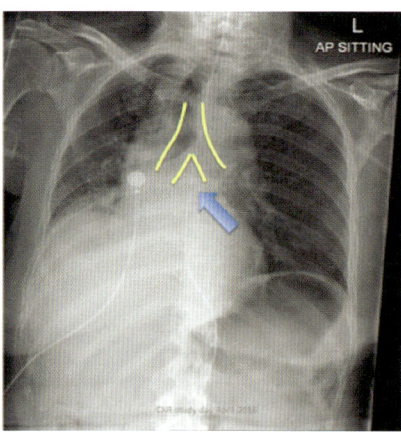

Figure 9.3 Does it bisect the carina?

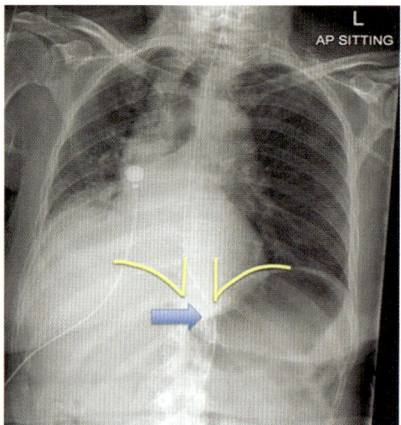

Figure 9.4 Does it cross the diaphragm in the midline?

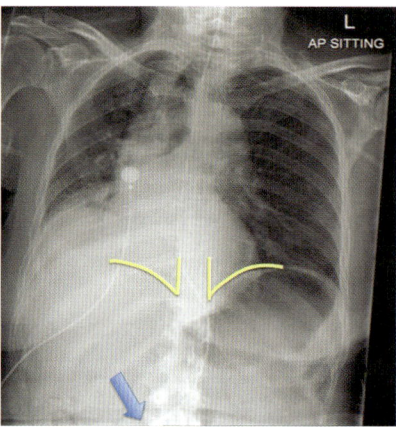

Figure 9.5 Does it pass at least 5cm below the diaphragm?

Other Trusts' initiatives on NG tubes vary, from radiographer reporters to radiologists reporting on all NG chest x-rays either immediately or within a specified timeframe. Only a few Trusts have radiographers specifically commenting on the position of the NG tube on the chest x-ray.

Central venous pressure (CVP) line

The CVP is a very common route for venous access; it may be used for fluid infusion or nutrition or drug administration, and also for monitoring right atrial pressure. The tip of the catheter should be optimally placed in the superior vena cava. On the AP chest image, the tip of the catheter should be 1–4cm below the medial aspect of the right clavicle.

Valves are present in the jugular and subclavian veins, and the tip of the CVP line must be distal to the valves in order to read atrial pressure accurately. The route of the CVP line to the superior vena cava can be either via the subclavian vein or jugular vein. The last valve in the subclavian vein is 2cm proximal to its junction with the internal jugular vein, and the last valve in the internal jugular vein is approximately 2.5cm above its junction with the subclavian vein. The brachiocephalic and superior vena cava do not contain valves (De Lacey *et al.* 2008, Karthik 2013, Mettler 1996, Tortora & Anagnostakos 1990).

The CVP tip may sometimes turn up into the jugular vein, if the route is via the subclavian vein; or it may sometimes cross the midline into the opposite subclavian vein. If the CVP line is too high, it can result in inaccurate readings of atrial pressure; if it is too low and in the right atrium, it can lead to cardiac arrhythmia. Other complications can be caused by the CVP line perforating the vessel wall, leading to pneumothorax, fluid in the mediastinum or pleural space, and/or nerve injury – e.g. brachial plexus (Chapman & Nakielny 1992, Karthik 2013).

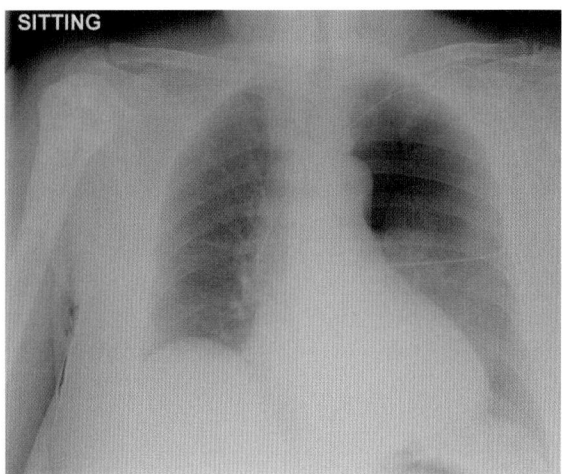

Figure 9.6 Left pneumothorax due to left subclavian line insertion

The Swan-Ganz or pulmonary artery catheter

A Swan-Ganz catheter is usually placed to monitor cardiac or pulmonary arterial pressures, to distinguish between cardiac and non-cardiac pulmonary oedema. The usefulness of these catheters is the subject of debate, as it is unclear whether or not they improve patient outcome (Binnay et al. 2005, Shure 2006, Finfer & Delaney 2006); however, they are still utilised so we should know where they should best be positioned.

The normal course is almost circular, down the superior vena cava, through the right atrium and ventricle and out into the main pulmonary and peripheral pulmonary arteries. The tip should therefore be optimally positioned between the main pulmonary artery and the interlobar arteries; and the tip should not extend more than 2cm beyond the mediastinal shadow. If the tip migrates too far, it can cause pulmonary infarct; if the tip is too proximal in the right ventricle, it can lead to arrhythmia.

Mettler (1996) comments on another route used for the Swan-Ganz catheter, via the inguinal area. In this case the catheter follows an S-curve, from the inferior vena cava into the right atrium and right ventricle and into the pulmonary artery. This is a much less common route than the one previously described but results in the same complications if misplaced.

Pleural drainage tube

These drainage tubes are normally placed to evacuate a pneumothorax or drain a pleural fluid collection. They are relatively large bore and inserted between the ribs in the mid or lower lateral chest. The tube has side holes which should be within the chest cavity, not in the soft tissues of the chest wall. If the tube is misplaced, with the side holes in the soft tissues of the chest wall, this will result in air leaking into the soft tissues and soft tissue emphysema. The tip of the drainage tube should therefore not abut the mediastinum or have a kink in it. If the patient is supine in the ICU, and the tube is placed posteriorly, it will have difficulty reducing the pneumothorax because the air will collect anteriorly, due to the patient's supine position (Karthik 2013, Mettler 1996).

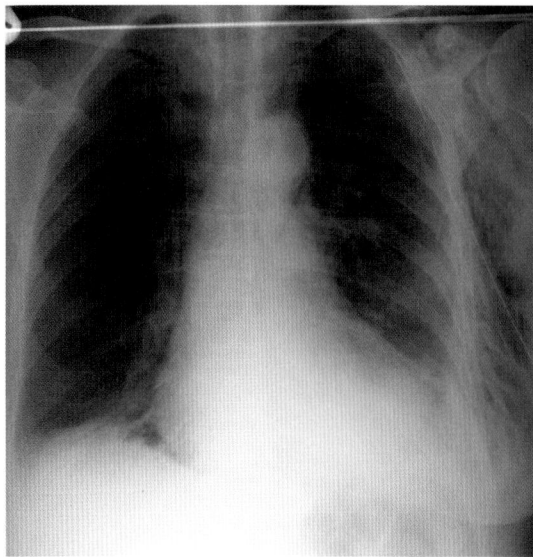

Figure 9.7 Air leak, due to last drainage hole being extra-thoracic

Nasoenteric tube

These are feeding tubes and the optimum position for the tip is distal to the pyloric sphincter. As the tube is thin and flexible, it can coil in the pharynx, oesophagus or stomach; or it can enter the trachea and right bronchus, leading to lobar collapse.

Tracheostomy tube

This type of tube should lie within the trachea. The walls of the tube are parallel to the walls of the trachea, the tip lying several centimetres above the carina, with the inflated cuff not bulging the tracheal walls. If widening of the mediastinum is demonstrated on the chest image, it may be due to a haematoma (resulting from the tracheostomy), although there is a wide differential for a widened mediastinum.

Pacemakers

Chest x-rays are often taken following insertion of a pacemaker. At this early stage, the chest x-ray is often used to check for complications of the surgery, such as pneumothorax, pleural effusion, or (rarely) myocardial penetration, which is likely to occur if the electrode tip is within 3mm of the epicardial fat.

It is also important to check that the electrodes are in the right position (De Lacey et al. 2008, Karthik 2013, Mettler 1996):

- Atrial pacemaker – electrode tip in right atrial appendage
- Single chamber pacemaker – tip of ventricular lead is in apex of right ventricle
- Dual chamber pacemaker – electrode tip in right atrial appendage, and apex of right ventricle
- Biventricular pacemaker – third lead along the coronary sinus.

Often pacemakers will be seen on chest x-rays taken for unrelated reasons, but an x-ray is still required to check the pacemaker electrodes are in the correct places, as well as looking for broken leads, and overlong or tight leads (which may move or break).

There are several types of pacing systems, which may be identified on a chest x-ray: single chamber, dual chamber, biventricular and implantable cardioverter defibrillators (ICDs). Complications can include mal-positioning (which occurs in 3–14% of patients) and myocardial perforation (where the tip of the lead projects beyond the heart border).

A single-chamber pacemaker can be of either the right atrium or ventricle, whereas a dual-chamber is of both the right atrium and ventricle and attempts to synchronise the two systems. In right atrial pacing, a J-shaped lead is manipulated into the right atrial appendage and is pulled upwards, embedding near the sino-atrial (SA) node. The lead tip points upwards and medially on the PA projection and upward anteriorly on the lateral projection. In right ventricular pacing, the tip of the lead is at the right ventricular apex. Radiographically, on the PA chest x-ray, it should be seen medial to the apex; whereas on the lateral projection it will be seen behind the sternum, immediately above the anterior costophrenic sulcus, inferior and posterior to the subpericardial fat stripe (Chen 1997).

Biventricular pacing involves pacing the right heart as described above, with an additional lead pacing the left heart via the coronary sinus. This enables access to the left heart via the safer, low-pressure right heart. The electrode may be seen in any of the tributaries of the coronary sinus but typically lies in the great or middle cardiac veins. Radiographically the lead can be seen to track to the left, posteriorly and superiorly (Chen 1997).

ICDs are used to manage specific ventricular dysrhythmias with a single lead that is radiographically similar to a single-chamber pacemaker but with a larger diameter. The lead goes with the venous flow into the right atrium, through the tricuspid valve and into the right ventricle. Pacing of the right heart is sufficient to cause contraction of the entire heart (Cooper & Kay 2008).

ICDs recognise and attempt to manage ventricular arrhythmias. Second-generation devices provide cardioversion (restoration of sinus rhythm by delivering a synchronised low-energy shock or pulse) in addition to the high-energy shocks. Third generation devices offer tiered therapy with anti-tachycardia pacing, programmable low-energy cardioversion, high-energy defibrillation and back-up bradycardia pacing (Moses *et al.* 2000).

Today some pacemakers are designed to be compatible with MRI, so a chest image may be taken to check the type of pacemaker. In those that are compatible with MRI, what looks like a spring is visualised in the pacemaker box.

Conclusion

There are many tubes and lines that may be found on the chest x-ray, often on patients in the ICU. Malpositioning may be fatal so knowing where tubes and lines should be positioned is imperative when viewing/reporting the chest image. This chapter has reviewed the most commonly found lines and tubes. However, there are some more rarely seen tubes and lines (such as the Doppler ultrasound probe for monitoring cardiac output) which have not been included.

When x-raying a patient's chest with multiple tubes and lines, you should try not to have unnecessary jumbles of lines over the chest (ask the attendant nurse for assistance), as they may hide small pathology, particularly in the neonate/paediatric patient (for instance, subtle rib fracture may be evidence of non-accidental injury). Extraneous tubes and lines will also make the job of assessing the correct position of lines and tubes even more difficult.

Key points to remember

- *When assessing a chest x-ray with multiple lines, take extra care to check that all the lines are correctly positioned, not just the one the clinician is interested in at that moment.*
- *Know the normal positions of all the lines, tubes and pacemakers that are commonly found on a chest x-ray.*
- *Review the image for related complications of the line, e.g. pneumothorax, soft tissue emphysema and aspiration pneumonia.*
- *If a line is wrongly positioned, get in touch urgently with the referrer/ward as per your local protocols.*

IF IN DOUBT, ASK!

CHRONIC CHEST CONDITIONS

Introduction

As there are many chronic lung conditions, this chapter will only briefly review those conditions that may cause diffuse lung fibrosis and their radiographic appearances, followed by some information on chronic obstructive pulmonary disease (COPD). For further information, please refer to the many detailed texts on this subject.

Diffuse lung fibrosis is also known as fibrosing alveolitis. The known causes of fibrosing alveolitis are sarcoidosis, collagen diseases, pneumoconiosis and allergic alveolitis, but it is sometimes idiopathic. Each of these will be briefly discussed in turn. The content of this chapter is based on material gathered from the texts listed in the references and information obtained from consultant chest radiologists.

Idiopathic pulmonary fibrosis

This disease process results in thickening of the alveolar walls with fibrosis and desquamation. As the disease progresses, the alveolar walls may disintegrate, giving rise to so-called 'honeycomb' lung. The radiographic appearance starts with ill-defined shadowing at the lung bases and lack of definition of the vessel outlines. Later, nodules with connecting lines may be seen. As the disease progresses, the lung volume decreases and circular translucencies may be seen; this is the previously mentioned honeycomb lung. As the disease becomes severe, the heart and pulmonary arteries become enlarged due to pulmonary hypertension.

Radiation pneumonitis

Radiation pneumonitis may occur following radiotherapy for intrathoracic neoplasms and breast cancer. Its appearance may vary between individuals, but within a few weeks, ill-defined small shadows may be seen in the radiation field; sometimes this may develop into fibrosis, which will conform to the radiation field, but ignore the lobar boundaries of the lung.

Collagen vascular diseases

This group of diseases includes rheumatoid arthritis, systemic lupus erythematosus, dermatomyositis and Wegener's granulomatosis. All these diseases may affect the lungs but this is often secondary to involvement of other organs.

Rheumatoid lung
The most common finding with rheumatoid lung is a pleural effusion. Pulmonary fibrosis may occur and this is often indistinguishable from idiopathic fibrosing alveolitis. A finding often associated with rheumatoid lung is rounded granulomas in the periphery of the lung. These may be single or multiple, normally less than 3cm in size, and may cavitate and resolve. Coal miners with rheumatoid arthritis may suffer from Caplan's syndrome, which produces multiple granulomas in the lung.

Systemic lupus erythematosus
With this condition, the chest x-ray usually appears normal. The most common abnormality is pleural effusion and cardiac enlargement.

Sclerodermia and dermatomyositis
The classic feature of these conditions is basal reticulonodular shadows due to pulmonary fibrosis. Normally the fibrosis is confined to the lung bases.

Polyarteritis nodosa
Patchy consolidations, some of which may be infarcts, are a common feature of polyarteritis nodosa. The consolidations may be repetitive. Care needs to be taken with repetitive consolidations, as a lung tumour may also cause this.

Wegener's granulomatosis
With this condition, the lungs will demonstrate one or several well-defined consolidations or masses which may cavitate. These are most often found in the mid zone of the lung.

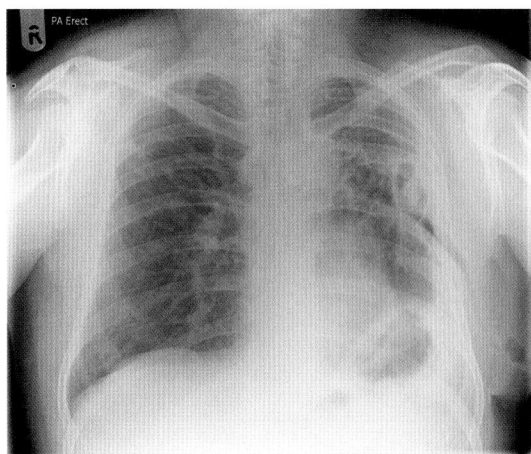

Figure 10.1 A patient with known advanced Wegener's granulomatosis of the left lung

Sarcoidosis
Sarcoidosis causes granulomas in many organs, one of which is the lungs. The diagnosis of sarcoidosis depends on the clinical, pathological and radiological findings.

The typical findings on the chest x-ray are:
- Hilar and paratracheal lymphadenopathy, normally bilaterally
- Reticulonodular shadowing/pulmonary fibrosis, maximal in the mid and upper zones.

The majority of patients with sarcoidosis of the chest have lymphadenopathy only, which sometimes clears without treatment and does not progress to pulmonary fibrosis. Such patients often have no chest symptoms. In rare cases, long-standing sarcoidosis may cause so-called 'eggshell' calcification of the hilar lymph nodes.

Pneumoconiosis

Pneumoconiosis is a group of lung diseases caused by the inhalation of a variety of dusts. Some of these inorganic mineral dusts (such as iron) are inert and, although they cause widespread small nodules, patients with siderosis have no symptoms and it does not progress to fibrosis. However, other types of pneumoconiosis (such as silicosis and coal miner's pneumoconiosis) are not inert and result in severe fibrosis in the lungs. Significant pulmonary fibrosis can occur with very small exposure to asbestos.

Coal miner's pneumoconiosis

Pneumoconiosis is due to dust retention, which leads to fibrosis. Radiographically, it is demonstrated as lots of small nodules in the lungs, starting in the mid and upper zones, and eventually involving all zones. This is called simple pneumoconiosis and often does not give rise to symptoms.

However, progressive massive fibrosis may supervene. It is demonstrated on the radiograph by homogenous shadows, often ovoid in shape, in the upper half of the lungs. These shadows may be unilateral or bilateral, with nodular shadowing in the rest of the lungs. Progressive massive fibrosis can cause breathlessness and cor pulmonale.

Asbestosis

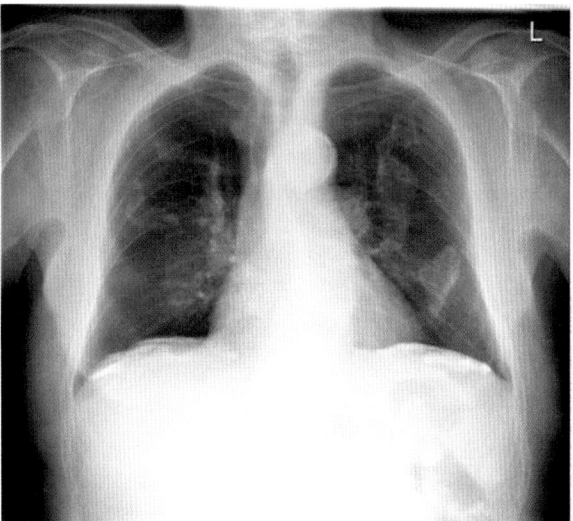

Figure 10.2 Patient with asbestosis, with large pleural plaques

Inhalation of asbestos fibres may lead to pleural fibrosis and calcification, as well as pulmonary fibrosis. The chest x-ray demonstrates initially localised plaques of pleural thickening, some of which will be calcified along the lateral chest wall and along the diaphragms. In asbestosis the pleural disease is bilateral – unlike other conditions with similar appearance, where it is unilateral. Often the costophrenic angles in asbestosis are clear of pleural disease, unlike other disease processes.

Pulmonary fibrosis is symmetrical, bilateral and maximal at the bases, resulting in fine reticulonodular shadowing, sometimes so fine that it has a hazy appearance (Chapman & Nakielny 1992, De Lacey et al. 2008, Mettler 1996, Weissleder 1997).

Determining the cause of fibrosis

Determining the cause of fibrosis can be difficult, but the distribution of the pulmonary shadowing may give a clue. In idiopathic pulmonary fibrosis, the lung shadowing is often more marked at the bases; whereas in sarcoidosis it is usually maximal in the mid zones. In scleroderma, lung changes are in the extreme lower zones; whereas in rheumatoid arthritis fibrosis the changes are either in the lower zones or uniformly distributed.

Personally, I find diagrammatic representations much easier to remember than written information. I have therefore put this information into diagrammatic form below, as an aide-memoire.

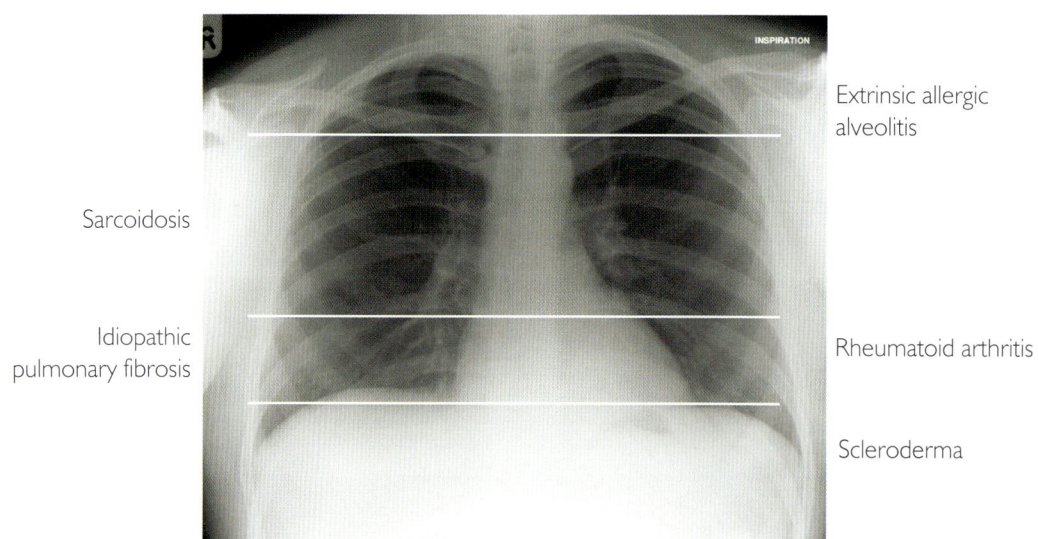

Figure 10.3 A diagrammatic representation of the distribution of diffuse lung fibrosis with different causes

The combination of pulmonary fibrosis with other signs can narrow the differential diagnosis even further:
- Past or present lymphadenopathy suggests sarcoidosis
- Coexistent conglomerate masses in the mid and upper zones are most likely to be silicosis or coal miner's pneumoconiosis
- Pleural thickening and calcification are most likely caused by asbestosis
- Past or present pleural effusions are suggestive of rheumatoid arthritis.

This section has given a quick overview of some of the causes of lung fibrosis, to assist in providing an accurate differential diagnosis when lung fibrosis is identified on a chest image.

Chronic obstructive pulmonary disease (COPD)

COPD is characterised by airflow obstruction that is not fully reversible and does not change over several months (Kaul 2007). It is an abnormal inflammatory response of the lung to noxious particles or gases, which is mainly caused by cigarette smoking (Hogg 2001, Devereux 2007). COPD is a condition that includes chronic bronchitis, emphysema and sometimes chronic asthma.

Devereux (2007) states that COPD was the fourth leading cause of death in the USA and Europe in 2007. Smoking is the main cause of COPD but there are other risk factors, including air pollution, prolonged exposure to dust and chemicals, and rare genetic causes.

Emphysema

Emphysema is defined as permanent enlargement of the air spaces distal to the terminal bronchioles, accompanied by destruction of their walls, but without obvious fibrosis (Kaul 2007). However, others comment that fibrosis may be present (Cottin 2005).

Emphysema can be classified according to its location. Panlobular emphysema leads to enlargement of all air spaces distal to the terminal bronchioles; whereas centrilobular emphysema involves the centriacinar respiratory bronchioles but spares the distal lung units.

Kazerooni (2001) divided the radiological appearances of emphysema into primary signs of lung destruction and secondary signs of hyperinflation. Destruction results in irregular radiolucency of the lungs, arterial depletion and thin-walled bullae, mainly demonstrated on CT. Bullae may enlarge and progress over months and years, resulting in displacement of vessels.

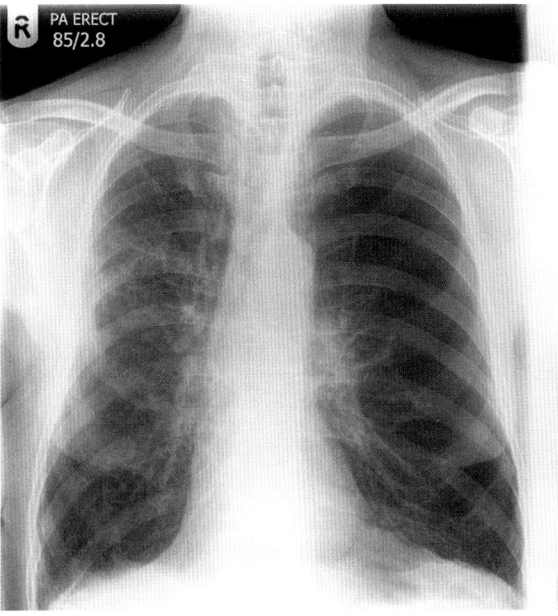

Figure 10.4 Large left-sided bullae

Chronic bronchitis

Chronic bronchitis is defined as a productive chronic cough lasting for three months, in two consecutive years (other causes having been excluded). It is caused by hypertrophy of the bronchial mucous glands and an abnormal increase in mucous production, leading to the bronchial walls becoming inflamed. This results in mucous plugging of the small airways which can lead to infection. A repeated cycle of repair and injury due to the inflammation can reduce the elastic recoil, resulting in air trapping. Grenier (2001) states that 21–30% of chronic bronchitis patients have a normal chest x-ray. However, some chest x-rays may demonstrate pulmonary hyperinflation, bronchial wall thickening, and increased lung markings.

Hyperinflation is demonstrated by reduced upward convection or even depression of the diaphragms. Other features of hyperinflation are an enlarged retrosternal clear space, narrowing of the transverse cardiac diameter and increased anterior posterior chest diameter – the so-called barrel chest.

Asthma

Grenier (2001) describes asthma as bronchial hyper-reactivity with varying degrees of obstruction. Its effects are reversible. It is predominantly an inflammatory process. Often the chest x-ray is normal.

Key points to remember

- *With chronic chest conditions, it is even more important to assess previous images and clinical details.*
- *Look for changes from previous images – is there new consolidation, etc.?*
- *Remember the combination of pulmonary fibrosis with other signs can narrow the differential diagnosis even further.*
- *Past or present lymphadenopathy suggests sarcoidosis.*
- *Coexistent conglomerate masses in the mid and upper zones are most likely to be silicosis or coal miner's pneumoconiosis*
- *Pleural thickening and calcification is most likely to be asbestosis*
- *Past or present pleural effusions are suggestive of rheumatoid arthritis.*

BE AWARE OF THE APPEARANCE OF EMPHYSEMA/COPD.

TUBERCULOSIS

Introduction

Tuberculosis (TB) is caused by the organism mycobacterium tuberculosis, and it can attack any part of the body. Pulmonary tuberculosis is the most common form and will be the focus of this chapter. TB can lie dormant in a person for many years, and an individual may never develop the disease. Alternatively, it may become active when their health deteriorates, or if their immune system is suppressed, or in old age.

An ancient disease, found in the spinal columns of Egyptian mummies, TB was identified in 460 BCE by Hippocrates as the most widespread disease in ancient Greece, and one that was almost always fatal.

TB spreads through the air from person to person; a person who is sick can spread the disease with a cough, but a symptom-free person, who is infected with tubercle bacilli, is not infectious.

TB is increasing in areas where human immunodeficiency virus (HIV) is endemic. The largest increase in TB cases worldwide is among people aged 25 to 44, the group most often affected by acquired immune deficiency syndrome (AIDS). TB is a common opportunistic infection among AIDS patients.

Babies, young children, the elderly, those with weak immune systems and people infected with HIV are at risk of developing TB. Ida (1995) and Wiwat (1999) list and discuss some of the diseases which put a person at risk of developing pulmonary TB, and those who are vulnerable to TB.

Patients are at risk of developing TB if they have:
- Diabetes mellitus
- Silicosis
- Cancer, leukaemia
- Substance abuse
- Severe kidney disease
- Malnutrition
- Heavy addiction to smoking
- Dependence on steroids.

The following factors make patients vulnerable to TB:
- Family and close contacts with active TB
- Being elderly
- Low income

- Poor access to healthcare
- Injecting illicit drugs
- Working in 'at risk' settings, e.g. prisons, nursing homes, shelters for homeless or drug treatment centres
- Being exposed to TB as a healthcare worker.

This chapter will continue to review TB, but now concentrating on the appearance of the chest x-ray; it will comment on primary tuberculosis and post-primary tuberculosis and signs that the disease is active.

Primary tuberculosis

Primary tuberculosis is the result of the first infection with mycobacterium tuberculosis and usually occurs in childhood. Post-primary TB, is thought to be a reinfection and usually occurs in adults.

In primary TB an area of consolidation, called the Ghon focus, develops in the periphery of the lungs, often in the mid or upper zones. The consolidation may be very small and is often accompanied by hilar or mediastinal lymph node enlargement. This combination of lymph adenopathy and pulmonary consolidation is known as the primary complex. The clinical features of the primary complex are often minimal and may go unrecognised; other patients may have a fever, cough and malaise. The primary complex then heals and calcifies; this calcification remains visible throughout life.

The infection may spread through the bronchial tree, leading to tuberculosis bronchopneumonia. On the chest x-ray, this will appear as patchy or lobar consolidation which may cavitate.

The infection may also spread via the bloodstream, resulting in miliary TB. The term miliary TB refers to the millet seed appearance of the nodules scattered throughout the lungs. These nodules are 0.5–2.0mm in diameter (De Lacey *et al.* 2008) and often mainly occur in the upper lobes. The primary complex is sometimes visible as well. Pleural effusions may also be present in primary TB.

Post-primary tuberculosis

The patient usually presents in adulthood with a cough, haemoptysis, weight loss malaise and night sweats. Post-primary TB is normally seen on the chest x-ray in the upper posterior portion of the chest as multiple small areas of consolidation. If the disease progresses, the consolidations enlarge and can cavitate. The infection may undergo partial or complete healing at any stage, resulting in fibrosis and calcification. Occasionally TB may present as lower or middle lobe bronchopneumonia. In some patients mediastinal and hilar adenopathy may be the only feature; this is more common in non-Caucasians.

As with primary TB, post-primary TB can spread, resulting in miliary TB and bronchopneumonia. Pleural effusions are commonly seen and, when they heal, they often leave permanent pleural thickening which may calcify.

The fungus Aspergillus fumigatus may colonise old tuberculous cavities, producing a fungal ball, called a mycetoma.

Is the TB active?

Ascertaining whether or not TB is active requires clinical investigation, and the decision is based on sputum tests and clinical findings. It is difficult to determine whether the disease is active from its appearance on a chest x-ray, as the presence of calcification does not exclude activity. Serial chest x-rays are required to assess activity. In general, if there is no development of new lesions, and no change in appearance for six months after completion of treatment, the disease is likely to be inactive (Armstrong & Wastie 1989).

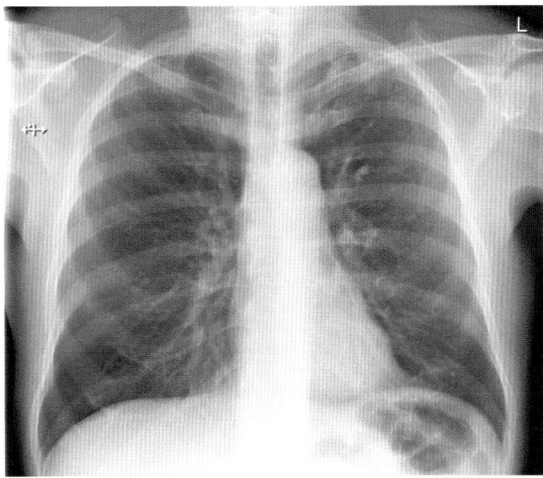

Figure 11.1 Probable TB demonstrated in the left apex in a 30-year-old patient; CT carried out to investigate further

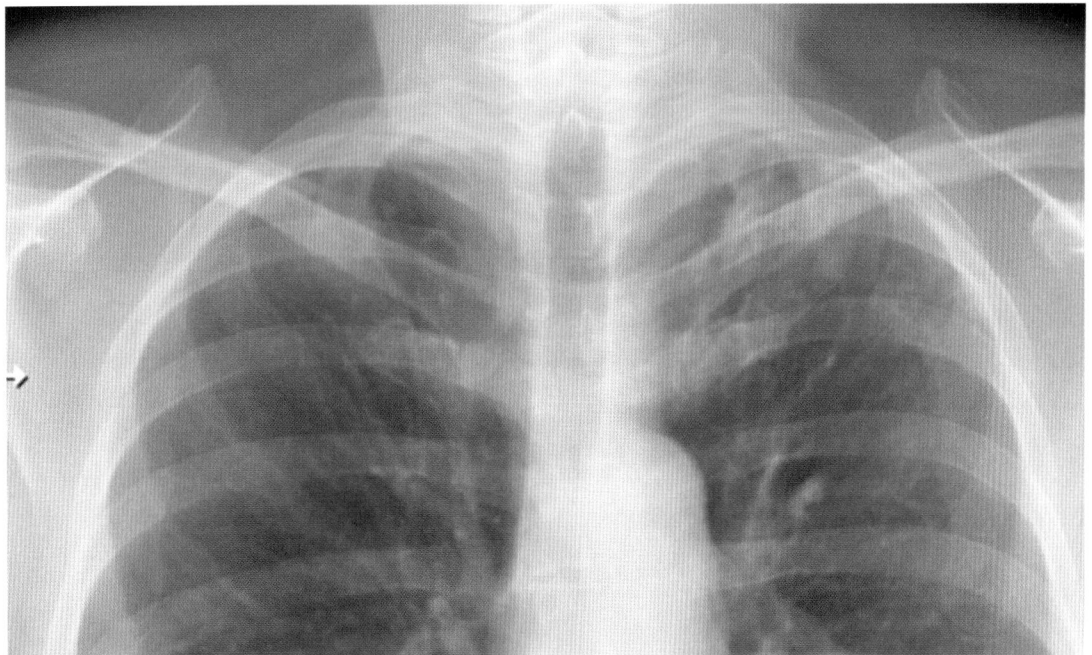

Figure 11.2 Probable TB in left apex of above patient – magnified view

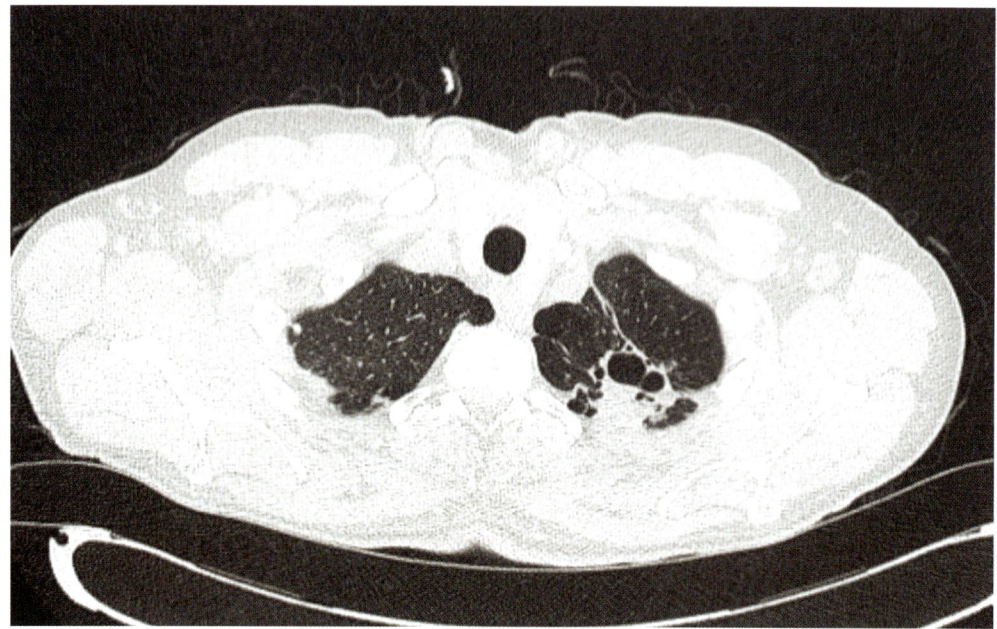

Figure 11.3 CT scan of the above patient helping to confirm left apical TB

De Lacey et al. (2008) contains a useful table commenting on active or inactive TB, which is summarised below.

Table 11.1 Active or inactive pulmonary TB

Active	Probably inactive
Cavitations	Marked calcification
Ill-defined shadows	Shadows well defined
Change from a previous chest x-ray, e.g. increased shadowing	No change on serial chest x-rays taken 6 months apart

Conclusion

In the UK, TB is found in the vulnerable groups listed in the introduction to this chapter. If the patient is from a vulnerable group, the clinician or chest reporter will often be suspicious that the appearances on the chest x-ray are a result of TB. However, 50 to 60 years ago in the UK, treatment of TB was not as advanced as it is today. Someone in this age group may therefore have been infected by the tubercle bacilli in childhood, and it may have lain dormant until the individual became immune suppressed or reached old age, at which point the disease became active.

People in the 50-plus age group are more likely to have lung cancer, and lung cancer and TB can have similar chest x-ray appearances in this age group, so this is something to be aware of. Clinical history, sputum tests and further radiological investigations (e.g. CT scanning) will lead to the correct diagnosis (Watson 2013).

When reviewing chest x-rays, it is therefore important always to bear in mind the appearance of pulmonary TB. so that it is diagnosed and treated at an early stage, before the patient infects anyone else.

Key points to remember

- *Be aware of the groups that are vulnerable to TB.*
- *Know the clinical signs of TB.*
- *Know the normal radiographic appearance of TB.*
- *Be aware of the appearance of miliary TB; compare with previous images. Are there any changes? Is the TB likely to be active?*
- *Remember that TB and lung cancer can look similar.*

12
60 Cases

Case 1

Clinical details: 80-year-old male, with persistent cough. Heavy smoker.

Describe what you can see.

What would your report suggest happens next?

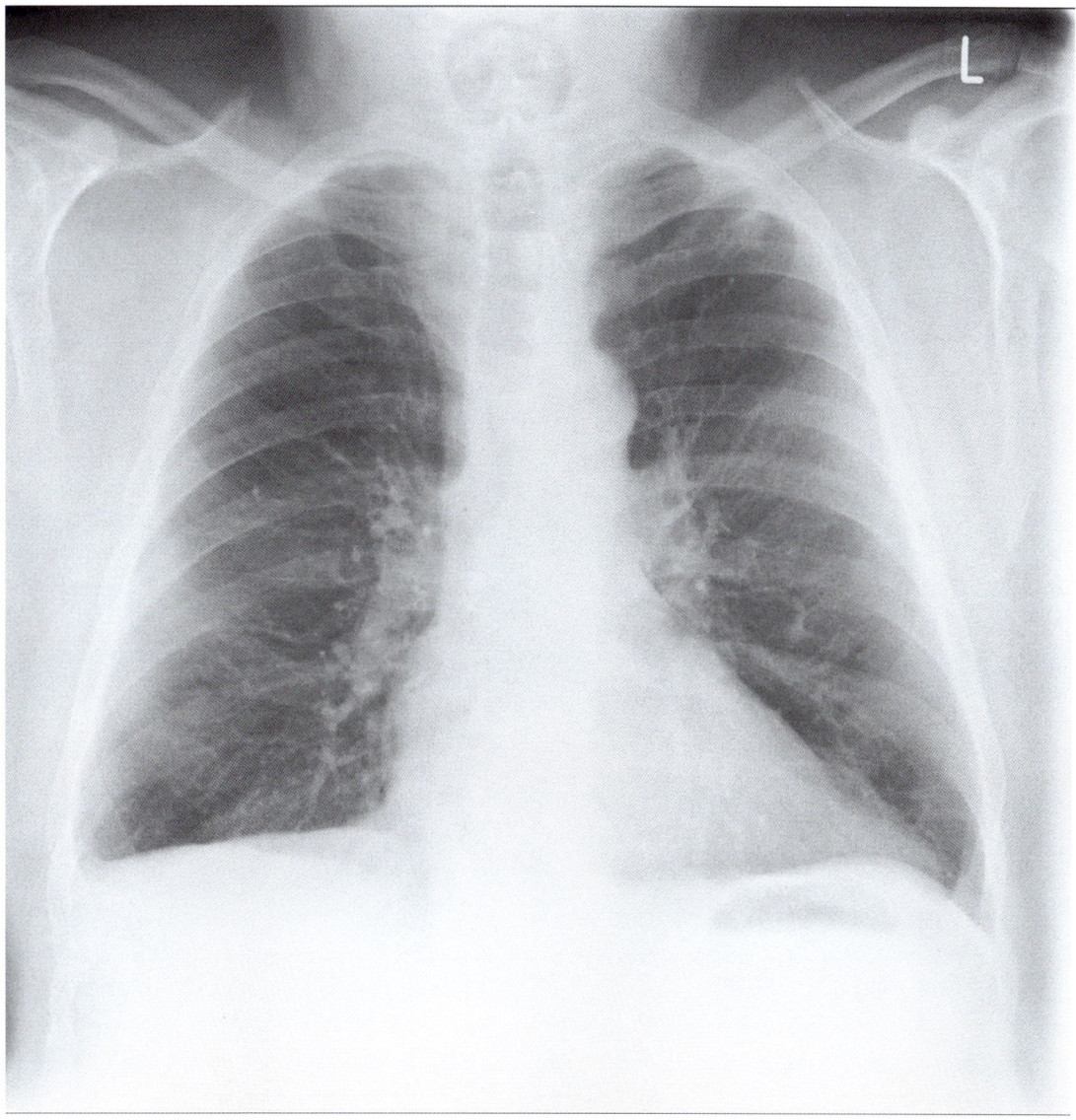

Figure 12.1

Answer to Case 1

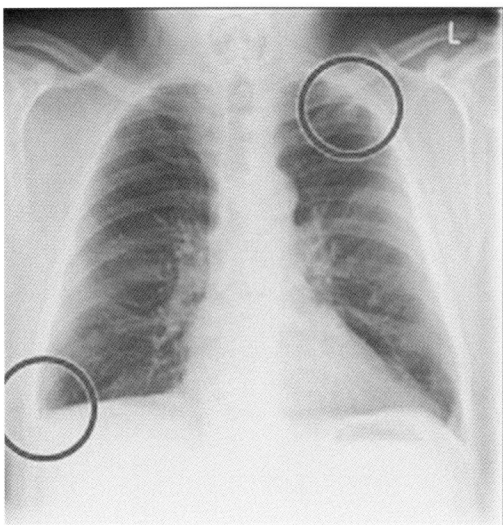

Figure 12.2

There is a small right-sided basal effusion. If there were bilateral small basal effusions and an enlarged heart and/or interstitial oedema, the conclusion would be heart failure. However, a unilateral basal effusion raises suspicion for lung cancer, unless there is another known cause for this (e.g. a fractured rib nearby).

A left upper zone mass can be seen close to the clavicle. Overlying scapula, and a lung density being over clavicle or rib, can make it difficult to visualise the lung density. Remember always to check the review areas, as this is where lung nodules can easily be overlooked. This lung density/nodule, considering the clinical patient details, is most likely to be lung cancer.

The patient should be referred to the lung cancer fast-track programme, and a high-resolution computed tomography (HRCT) scan should be performed. The patient should then be discussed at a multidisciplinary team (MDT) meeting.

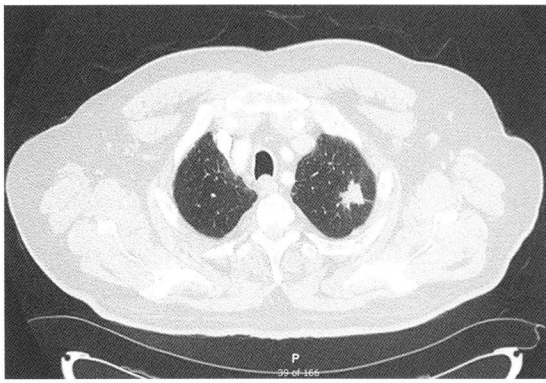

Figure 12.3

On CT, the cancer was staged as Stage IA (T1a, N0, M0) and treated with stereotactic ablative radiotherapy (SABR). Ideally, lung cancers should be picked up at this early stage to ensure the best outcome.

Case 2

Clinical details: known COPD, heavy smoker, persistent cough, 70-year-old male.

Describe what you can see.

What would your report suggest happens next?

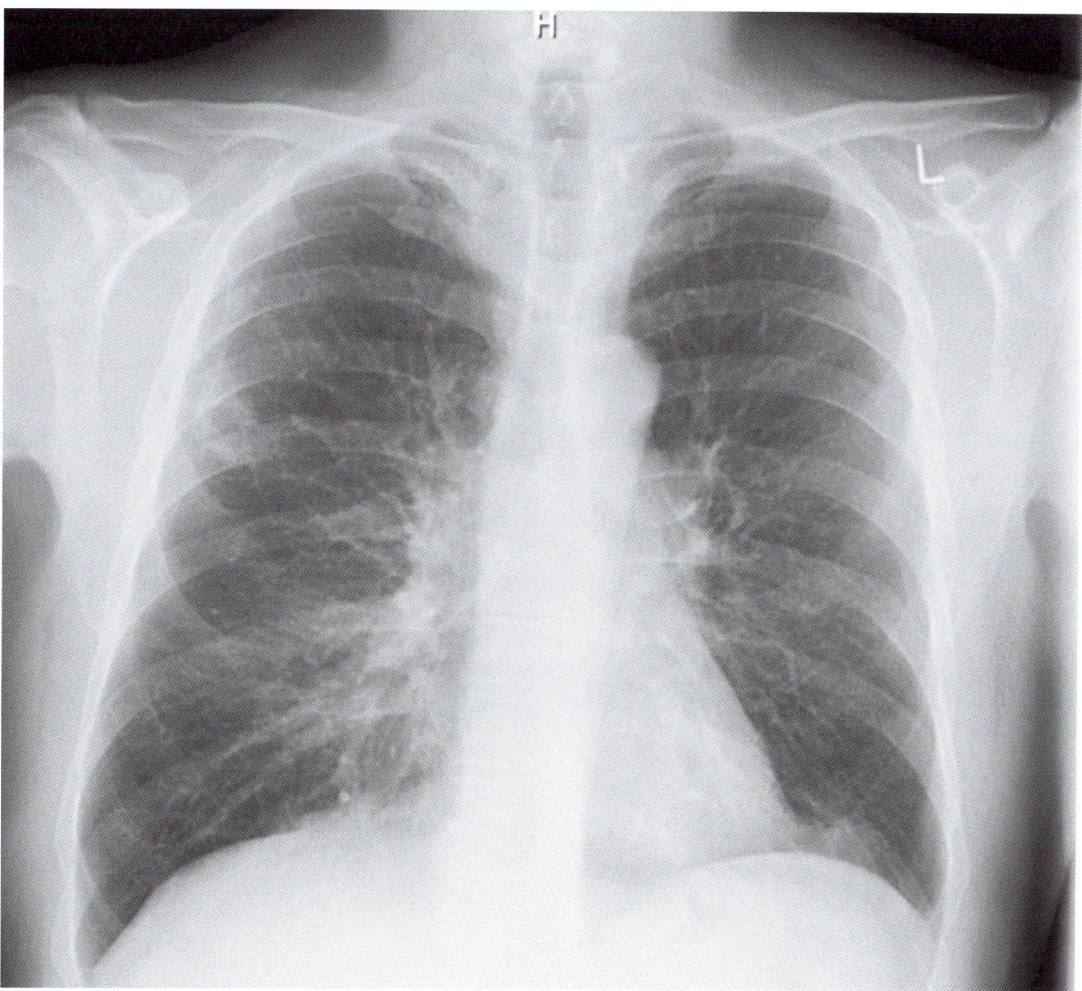

Figure 12.4

Answer to Case 2

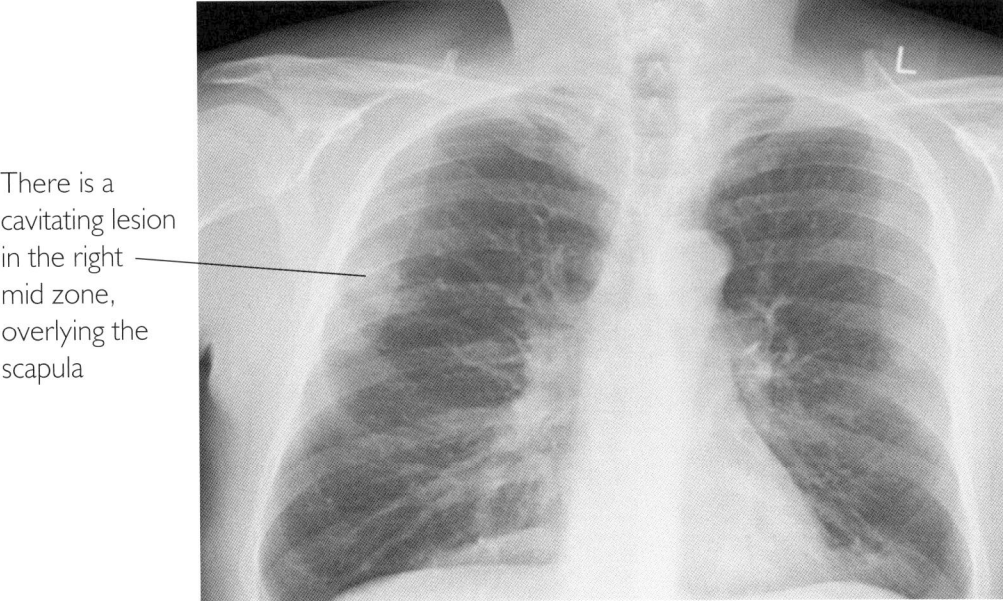

There is a cavitating lesion in the right mid zone, overlying the scapula

Figure 12.5

There is a cavitating lesion in the right mid zone overlying the scapula, again a difficult area to visualise. The right hilar also looks bulky. The patient was referred to the lung cancer fast-track programme and a CT performed.

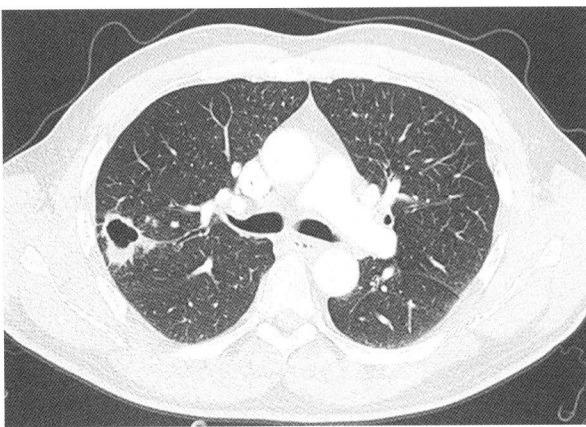

Figure 12.6

The staging from this CT and a PET scan was T2a pN0 pR0 and the diagnosis was an adeno-squamous carcinoma. Remember an adeno carcinoma is sometimes called 'the great pretender' as it can take on various disguises, and it can also cavitate.

Case 3

Clinical details: 65-year-old Accident and Emergency patient with increased difficulty in breathing.

Describe what you can see.
Does anything further need to be done?

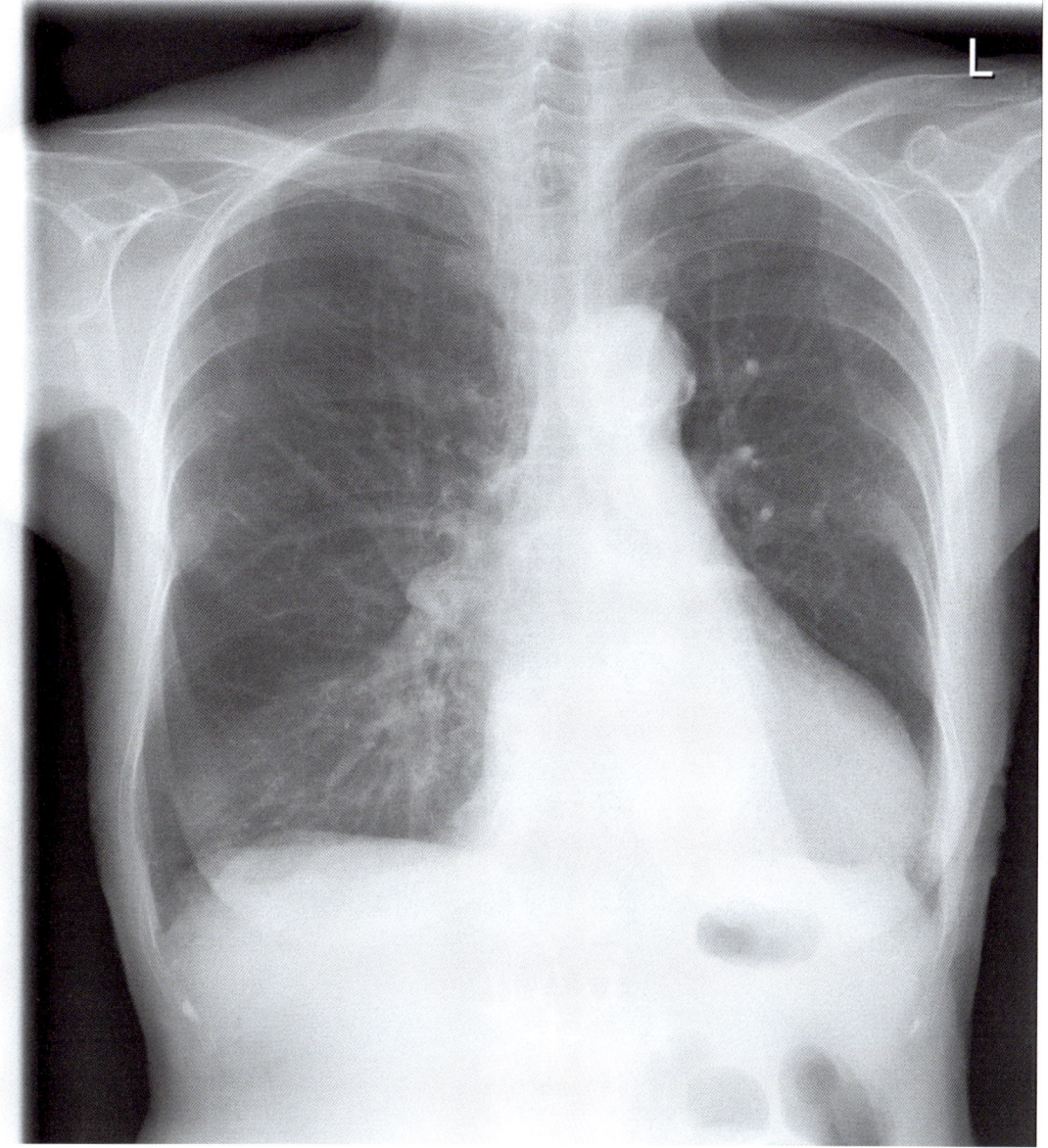

Figure 12.7

Answer to Case 3

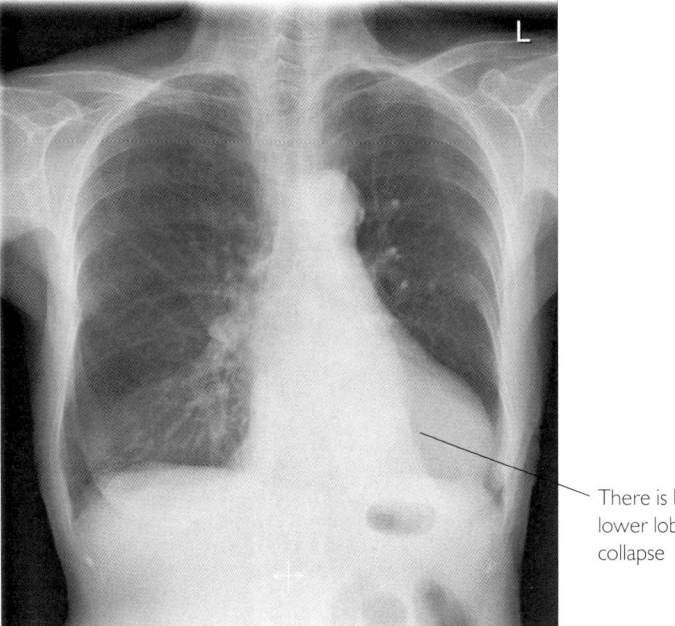

There is left lower lobe collapse

Figure 12.8

There is left lower lobe collapse demonstrated behind the heart. Remember Felson's silhouette sign (as described in Chapter 3). If you have forgotten about lung collapse, review Chapter 4 for examples of lung collapse. Left lower lobe collapse is often difficult to see and you need to review the area behind the heart carefully.

Lung collapse can be caused by a mucous plug or a lung nodule/lung mass. Further investigation is required to discover the reason behind the lung collapse; this normally involves a CT scan; bronchoscopy may also be required.

Case 4

Clinical details: 55-year-old with flu-like symptoms. Query chest infection?

Review the images.

Is there a chest infection or anything else?

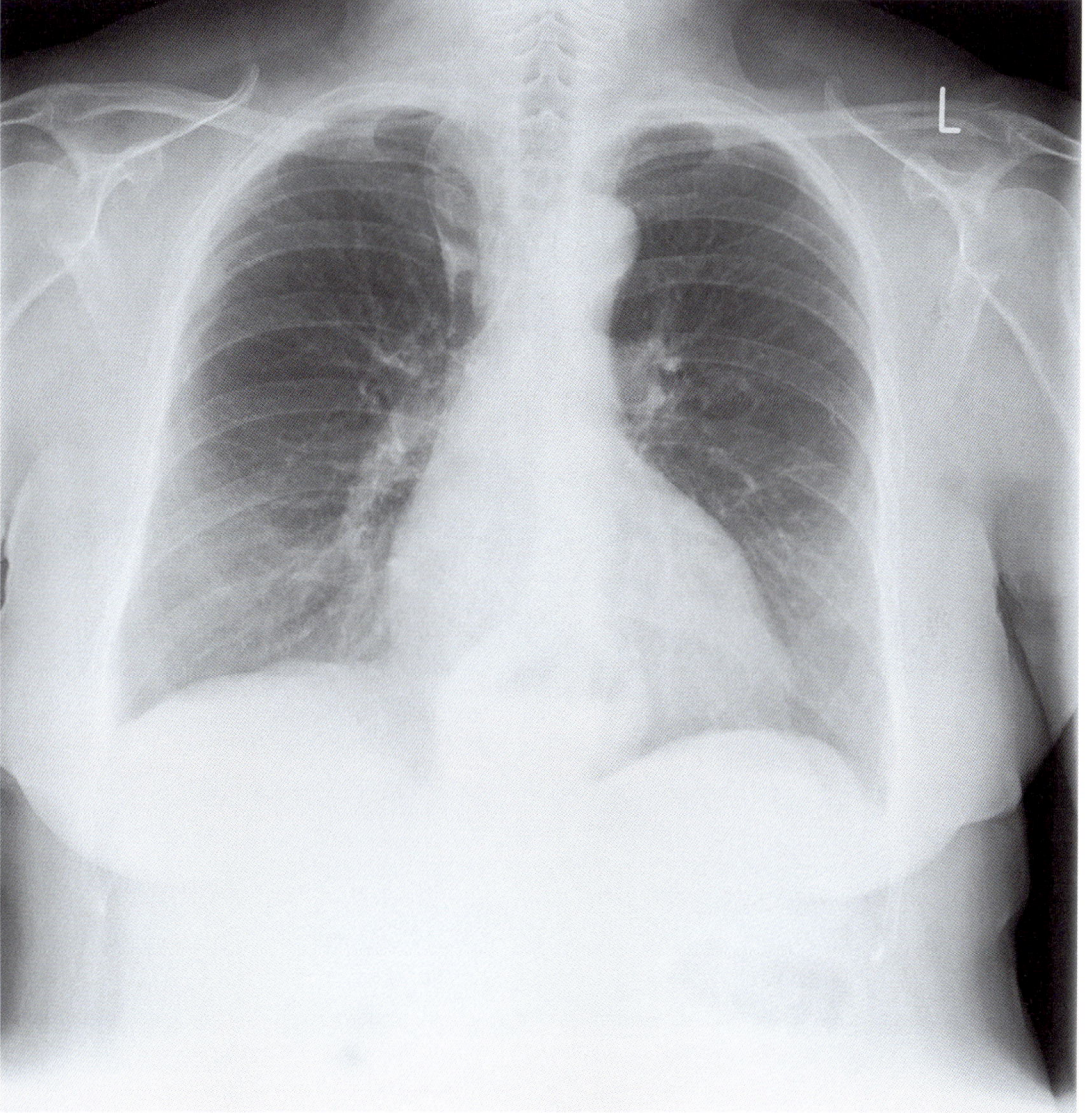

Figure 12.9

Answer to Case 4

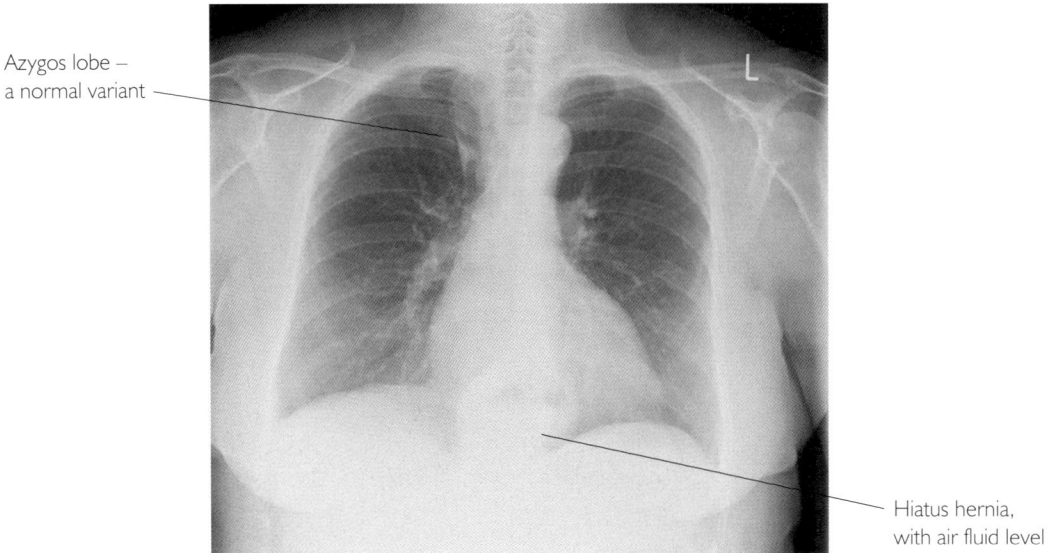

Figure 12.10

There is no sign of a chest infection, and no consolidation is demonstrated. Always answer the clinical question in your report, then continue to describe other identities. If follow-up is required, as in positive consolidation, state this clearly at the end of your report. If your report is quite long (for whatever reason), it is helpful to have a stated summary or conclusion, with the key point/s, at the end.

Also demonstrated on this image is an azygos lobe, which is a normal variant. Make sure you are aware of the appearance of normal variants, whether on a chest x-ray or a musculoskeletal (MSK) image. There is a hiatus hernia demonstrated behind the heart, with an air fluid level; so this is consistent with a hernia and not a mass at this site.

The heart size is at the upper border of normal, but there are no other signs of heart failure.

Case 5

Clinical details: elderly lady, now having increased difficulty breathing.

Describe what you can see.

What would you suggest happens next?

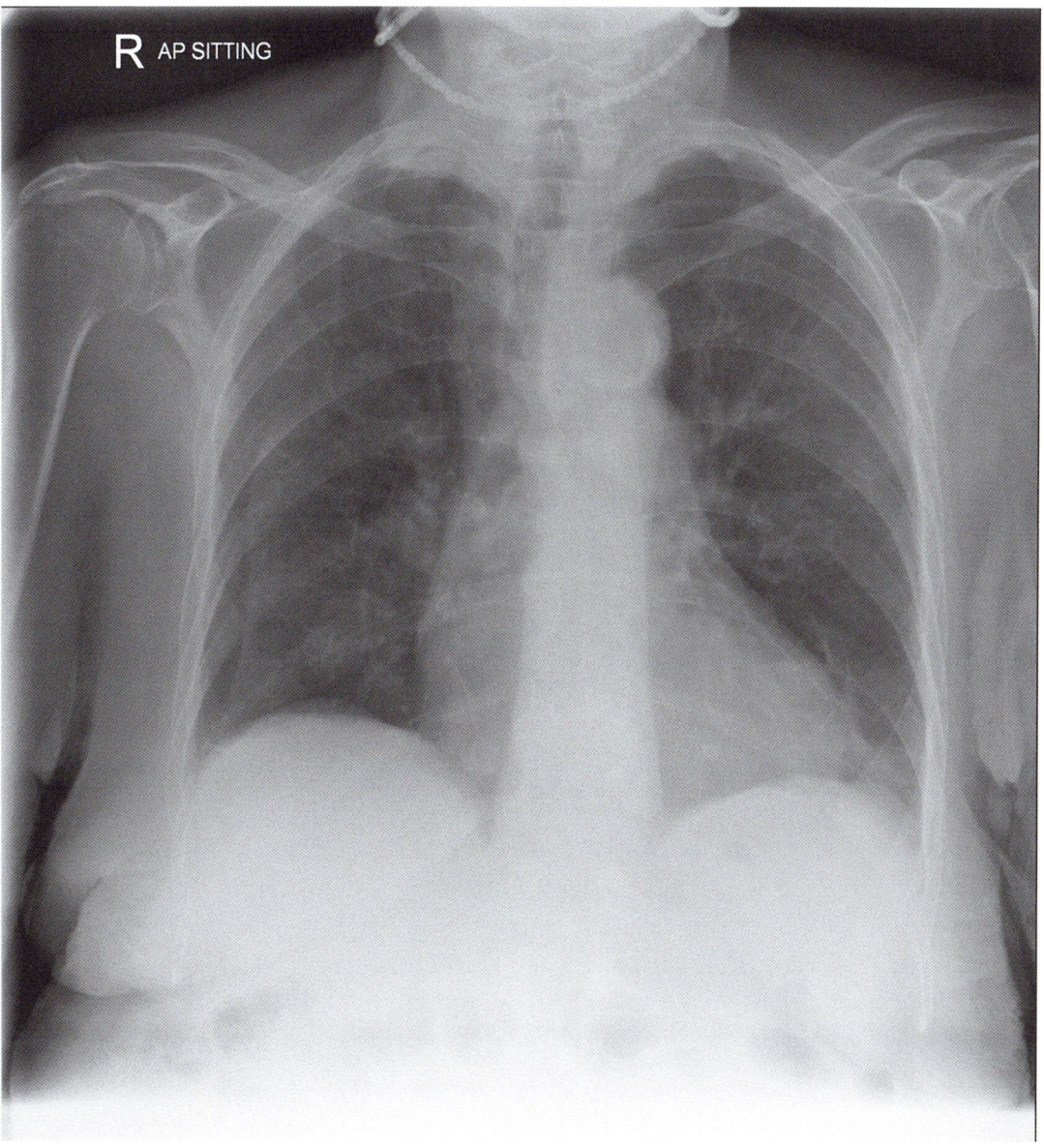

Figure 12.11

Answer to Case 5

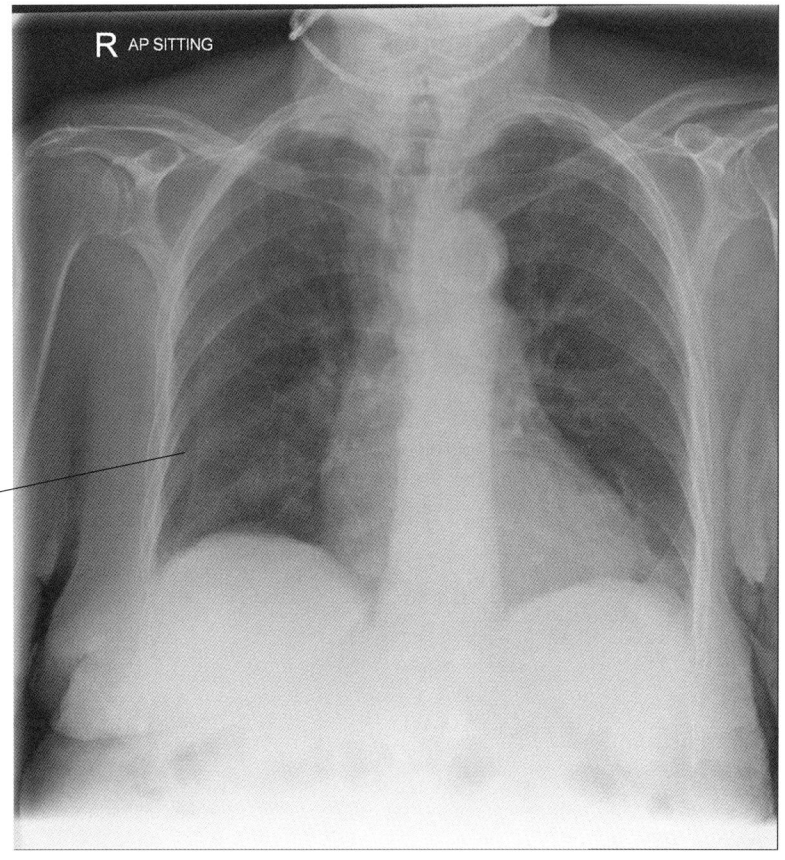

Line of a skin fold, *not* a pneumothorax; lung markings can be seen external to the line

Figure 12.12

The line at the lateral edge of the right lung is a skin fold, which can often be seen in elderly ladies who have lost a lot of weight. Be extremely careful not to mistake this for a pneumothorax (the lung marking can be visualised lateral to the skin fold). PACS is very useful in this case, as you can magnify/window this area to visualise it more clearly.

To answer the question at the beginning, state clearly in your report that this is a skin fold (not a pneumothorax), to prevent a chest drain mistakenly being put in. The patient is AP, sitting, and thus magnifying the heart. But, even allowing for this, the heart size is at the upper border of normal. The left base demonstrates interstitial oedema (Kerley Bs); appearances are consistent with heart failure.

Case 6

Clinical details: 30-year-old, with increased shortness of breath.

Describe what you see.

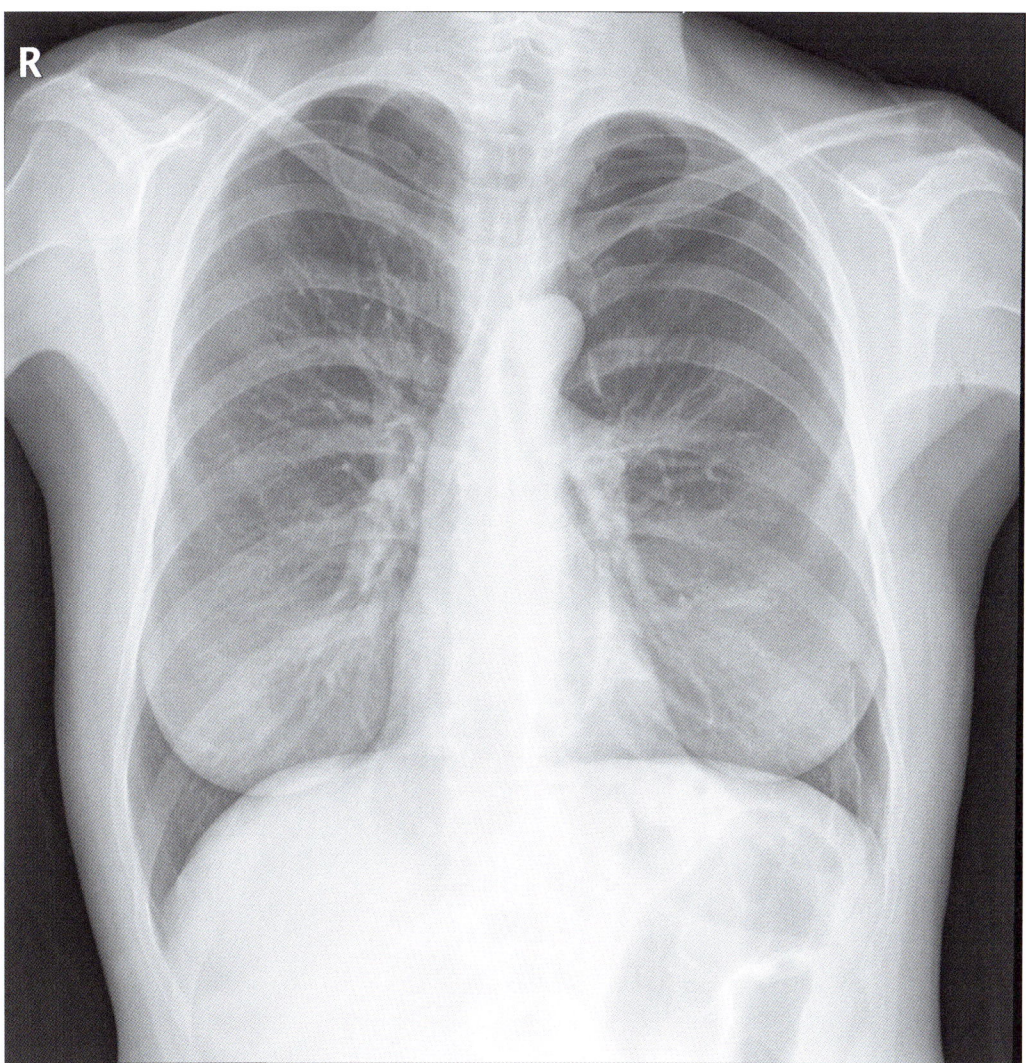

Figure 12.13

Answer to Case 6

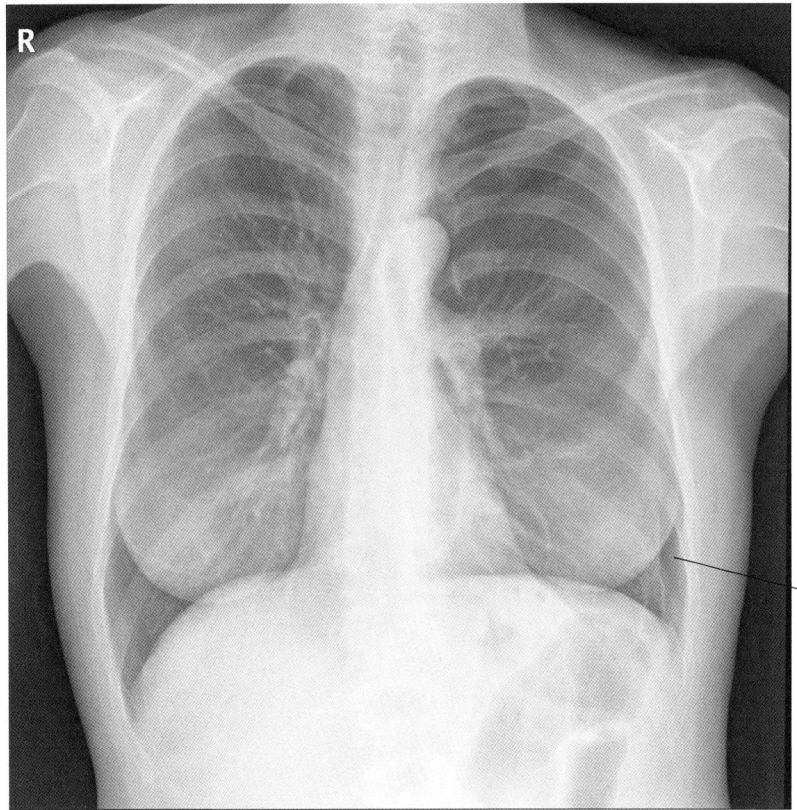

Line of a 4cm pneumothorax; there are no lung markings external to this line

Figure 12.14

This case demonstrates a left 4cm basal pneumothorax. This time no lung markings are demonstrated lateral to the line. The patient went on to have a chest drain inserted.

Case 7

Clinical details: patient has a chest drain in for a pneumothorax. This is a routine check chest x-ray after insertion of the chest drain. Is everything okay?

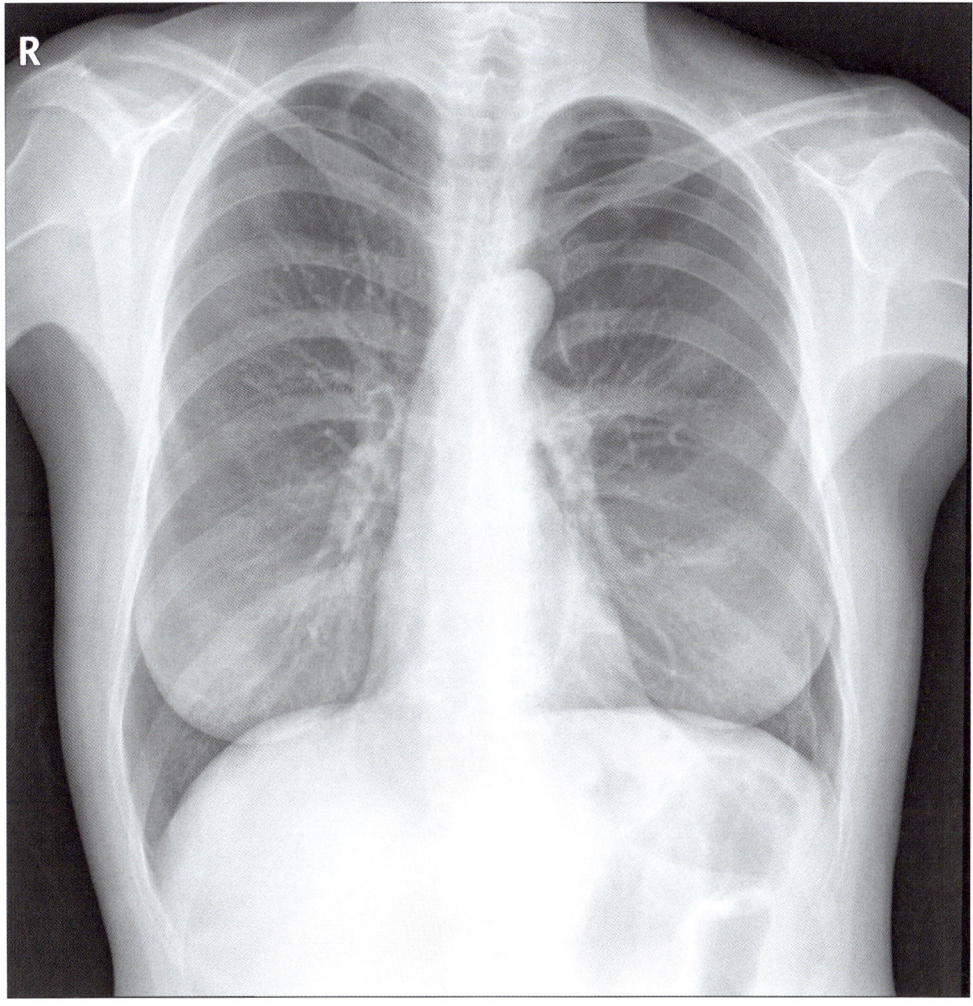

Figure 12.16

Answer to Case 7

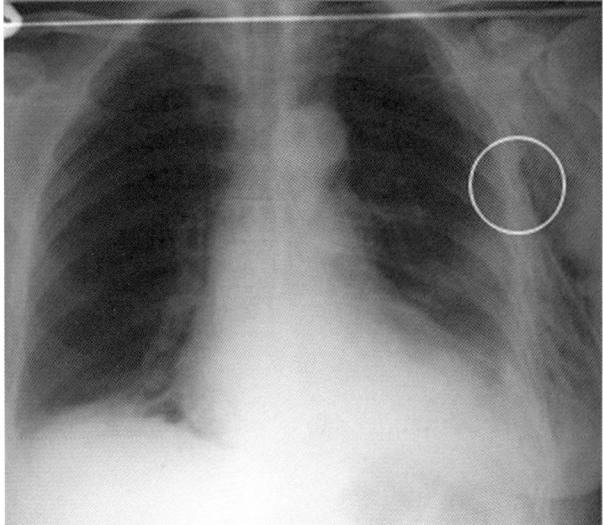

Figure 12.17

There is a continuing air leak due to the last hole in the chest drain being extra-thoracic, resulting in soft tissue emphysema. When reviewing chest images with chest drains in situ, you should not only be looking to see if the pneumothorax has decreased in size, but for other complications as well. In this case, only a small left apical pneumothorax remains.

Case 8

Clinical details: heavy smoker with known chronic lung condition. Query pneumothorax?

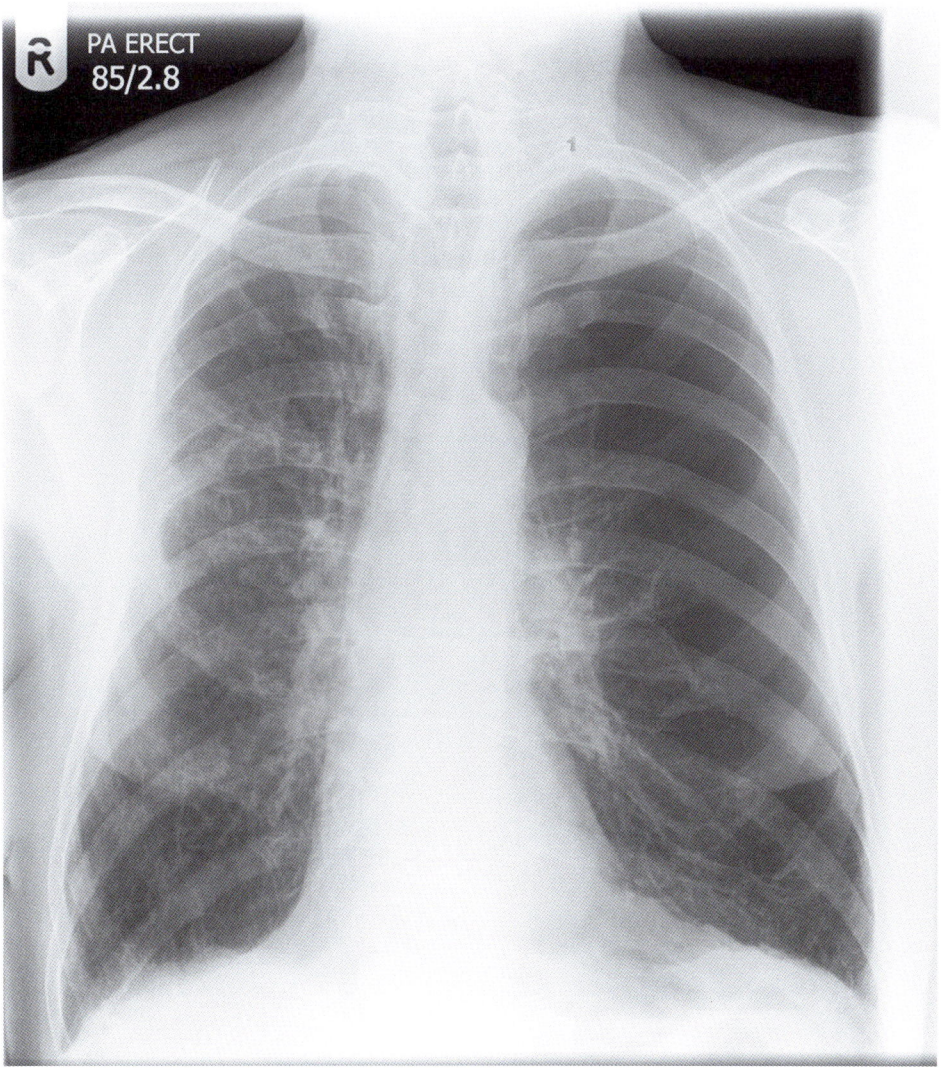

Figure 12.18

Answer to Case 8

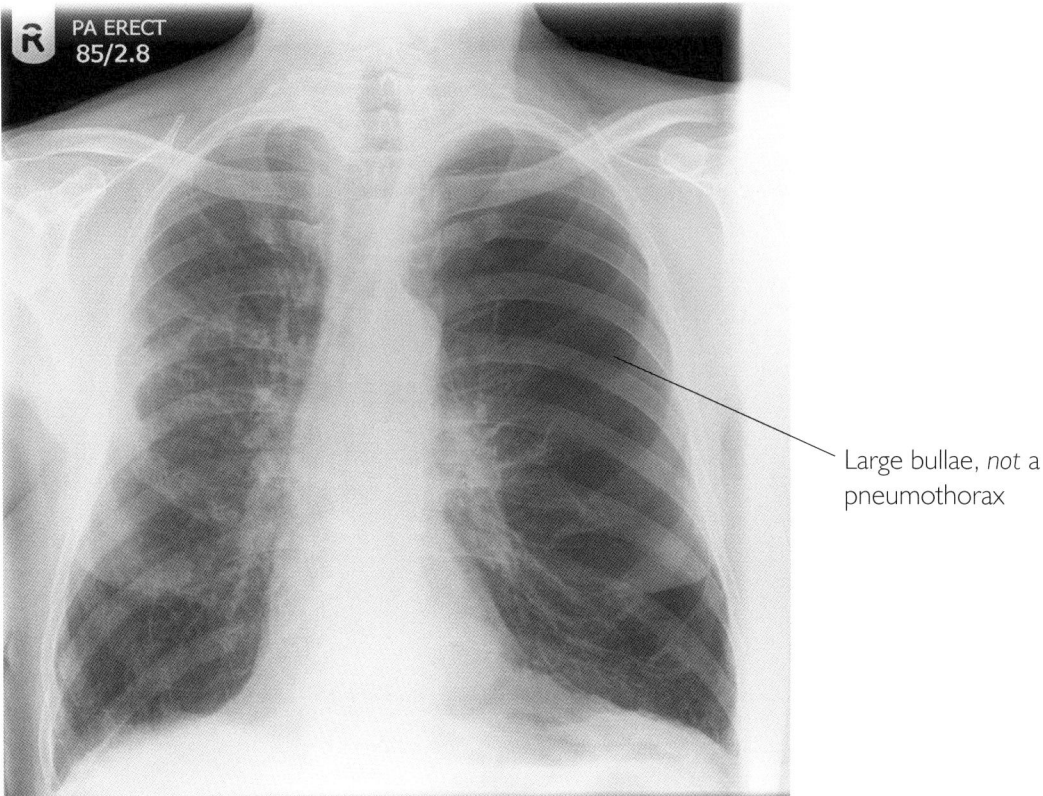

Large bullae, *not* a pneumothorax

Figure 12.19

The image demonstrates coarse lung markings, and over-inflated lungs with flattened diaphragms; the appearance is consistent with COPD. The left lung demonstrates a large bulla, with no lung markings within the bullae, but they are present external to this.

Case 9

Clinical details: 25-year-old female with cough and fever. Query chest infection?

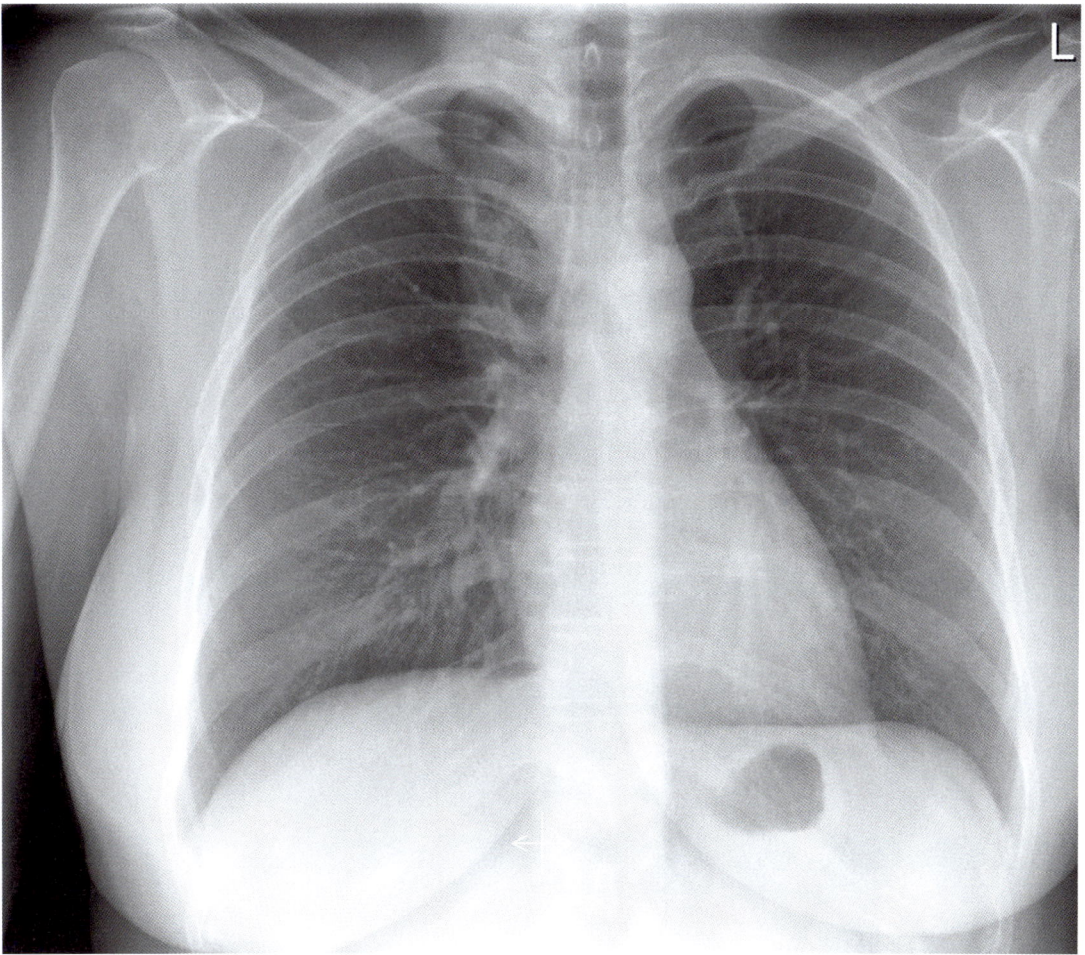

Figure 12.20

Answer to Case 9

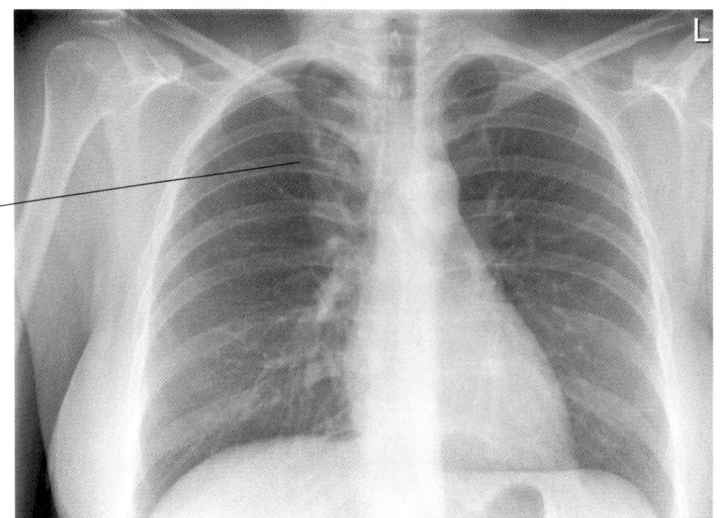

Appears to be a soft tissue mass in the upper mediastinum

Figure 12.21

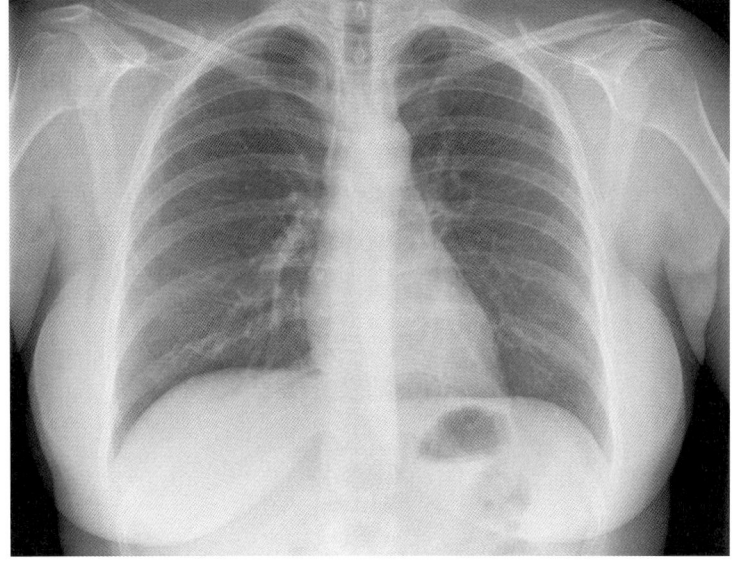

Figure 12.22
Repeat x-ray shows normal appearance

The first chest image is normal, apart from what appears to be a soft tissue shadow overlying the upper mediastinum. On closer inspection, it becomes clear that this is a hair plait. Digital imaging is much more sensitive than computerised radiography, and thick, plaited or wet hair will show up as a shadow on the chest image which can be misleading. The chest x-ray was repeated with the hair placed in a theatre cap (it is useful to have a box of these nearby, when carrying out chest x-rays).

The important point is to be careful when commenting on chest images and encourage radiographers to remove artefacts from the imaging site. Slogans on T-shirts will also be seen overlying the lungs on digital images if such T-shirts are not removed.

Case 10

Clinical details: unwell 26-year-old male, with cough and fever. Query chest infection?

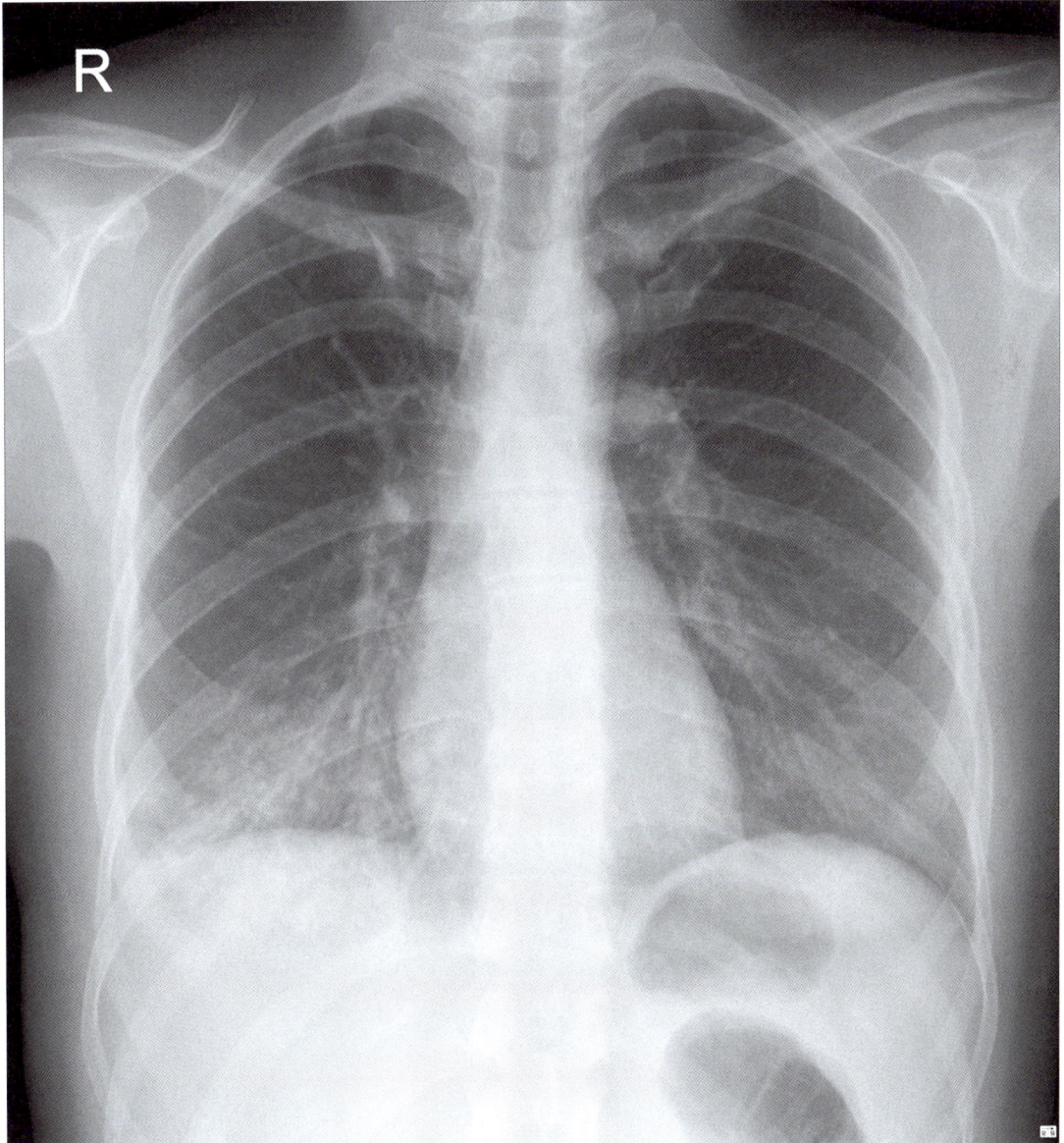

Figure 12.23

Answer to Case 10

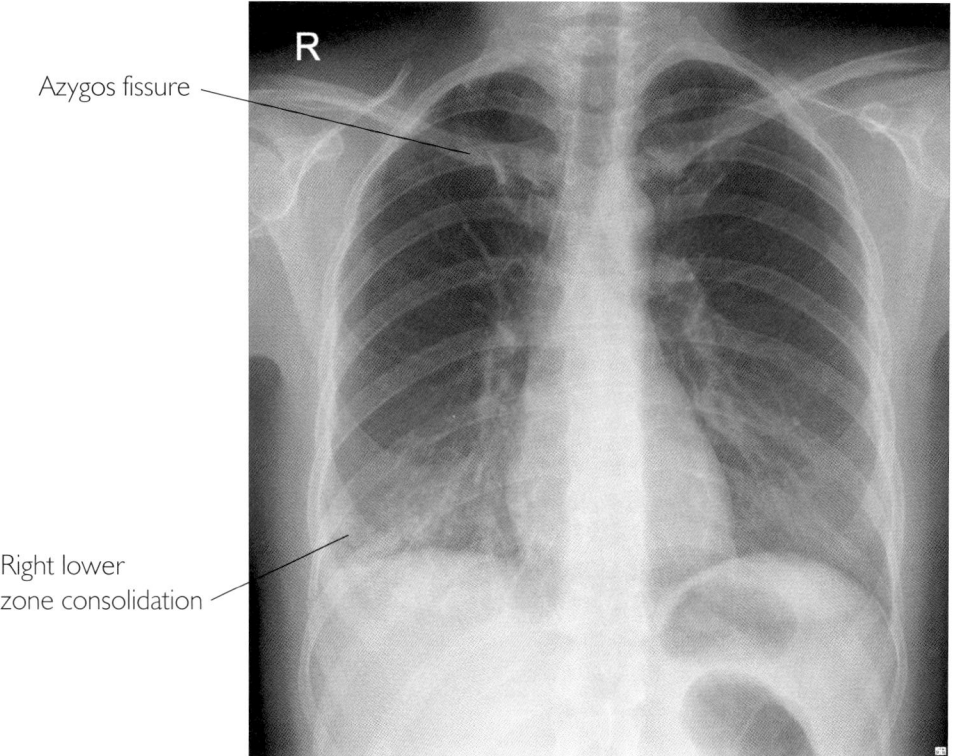

Figure 12.24

The image demonstrates right lower zone consolidation. Considering the patient's clinical details, this is most likely to be the result of an infective process. Suggest treat as infection, with repeat x-ray in 6–8 weeks to ensure resolution of appearances as per NICE guidelines.

This report answers the clinical question, and suggests appropriate follow-up. Notice how the consolidation has caused the right diaphragm to be ill defined, which is consistent with Felson's silhouette sign. There is also a normal variant demonstrated, an azygos fissure.

Case 11

Clinical details: 20-year-old road traffic collision patient. Difficulty breathing, with pain in left side of chest.

Comment on the image.

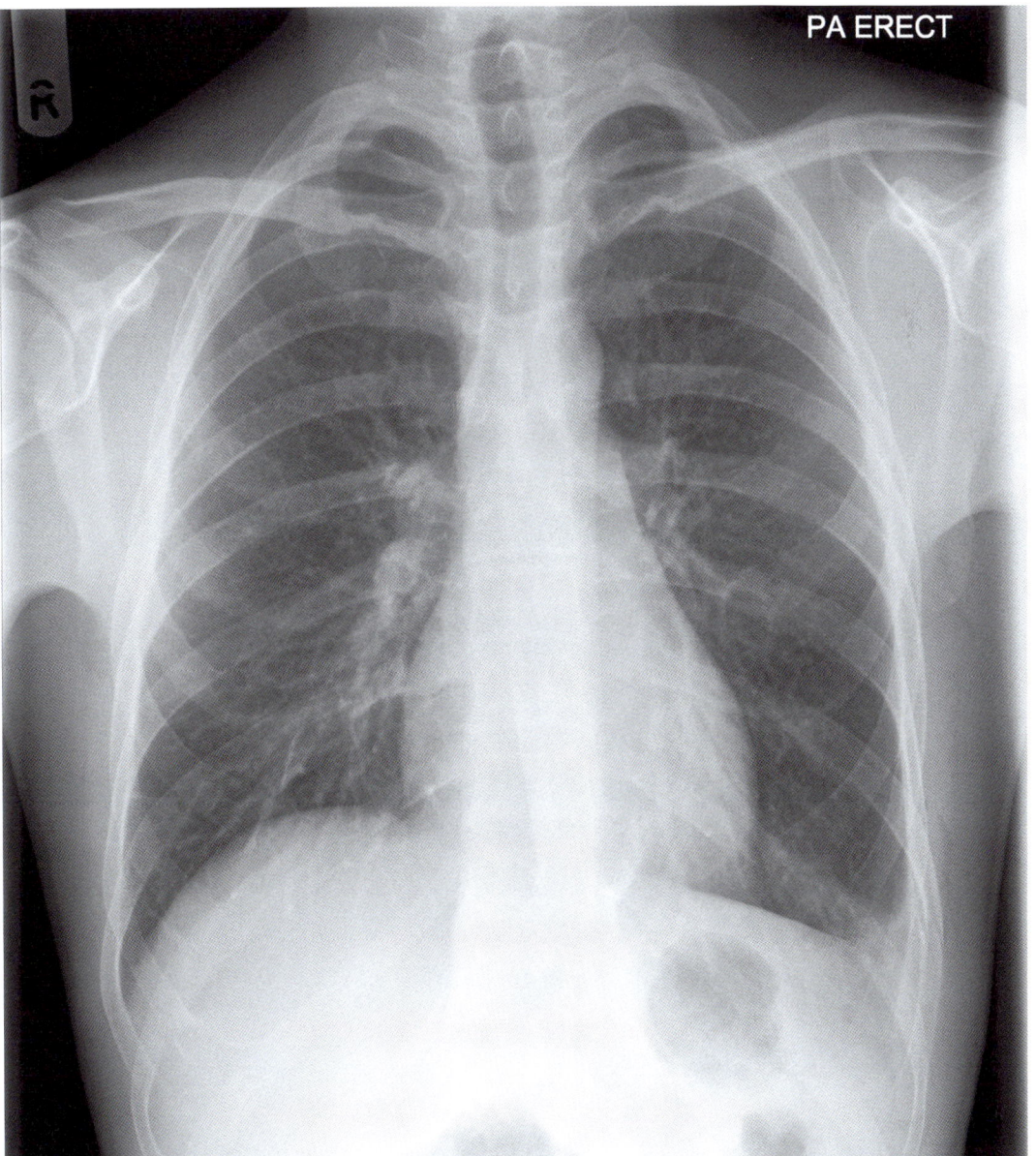

Figure 12.25

Answer to Case 11

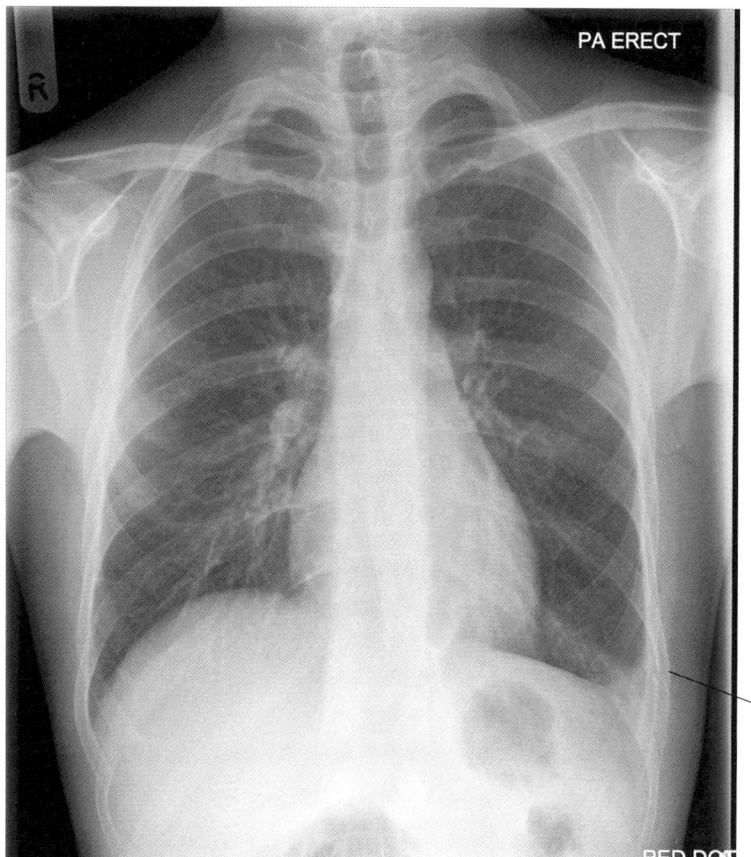

Fractured rib, with small haemothorax

Figure 12.26

There is a fracture of the left 9th posterior lateral rib, with a small haemothorax. No other bony injury is demonstrated; rest of chest x-ray normal.

Case 12

Clinical details: continuous cough, query consolidation?

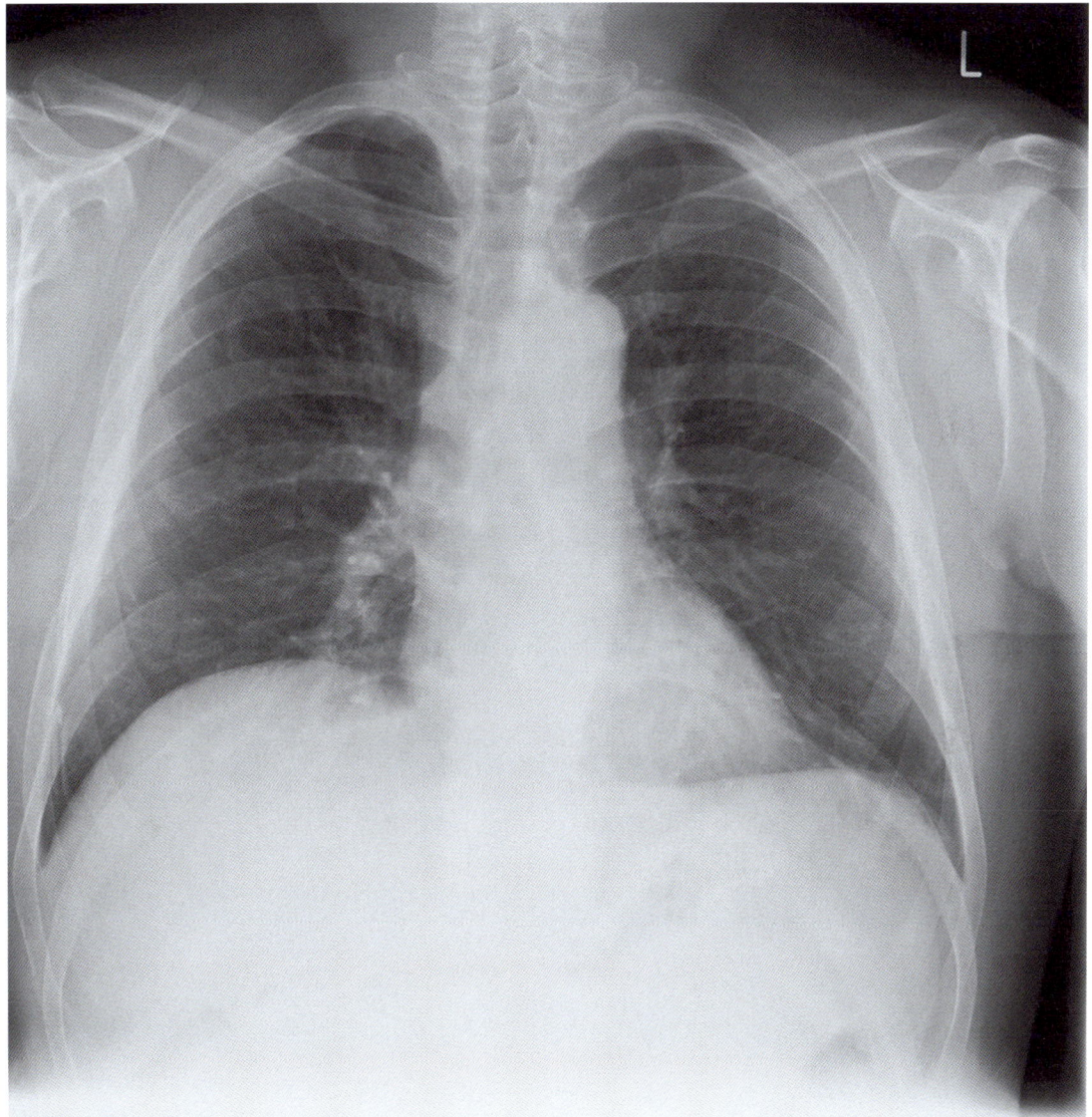

Figure 12.27

Answer to Case 12

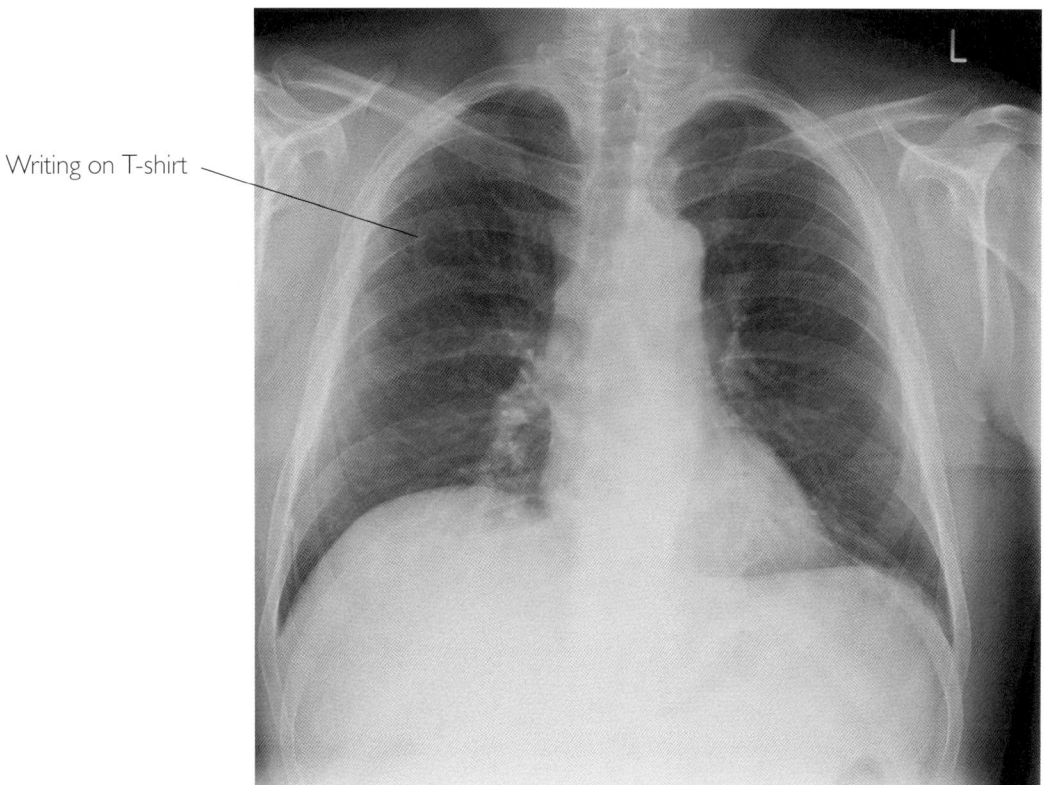

Figure 12.28

There is no consolidation present. The hilar does look slightly bulky, but this was consistent with previous images. The patient had been x-rayed with their T-shirt with writing on, which showed up on this digital image. This again demonstrates how artefacts can cause confusion. Patients should be x-rayed in an x-ray gown to prevent this.

Case 13

Clinical details: patient has severe difficulty breathing, in resuscitation room. What is causing this?

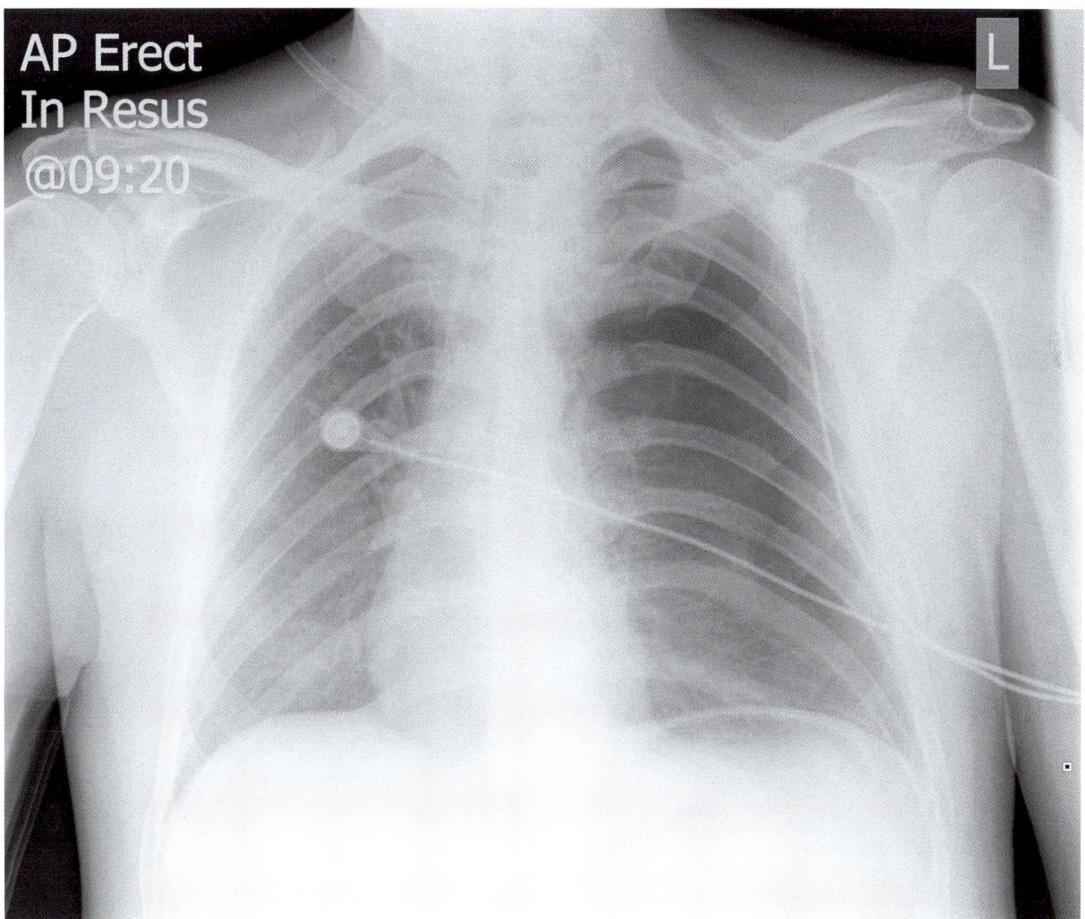

Figure 12.29

Answer to Case 13

There is a large left-sided tension pneumothorax, movement of the heart and mediastinal structures is demonstrated. A chest drain will be inserted.

Case 14

Clinical details: chest x-ray needed to check nasogastric (NG) tube position. Comment on this.

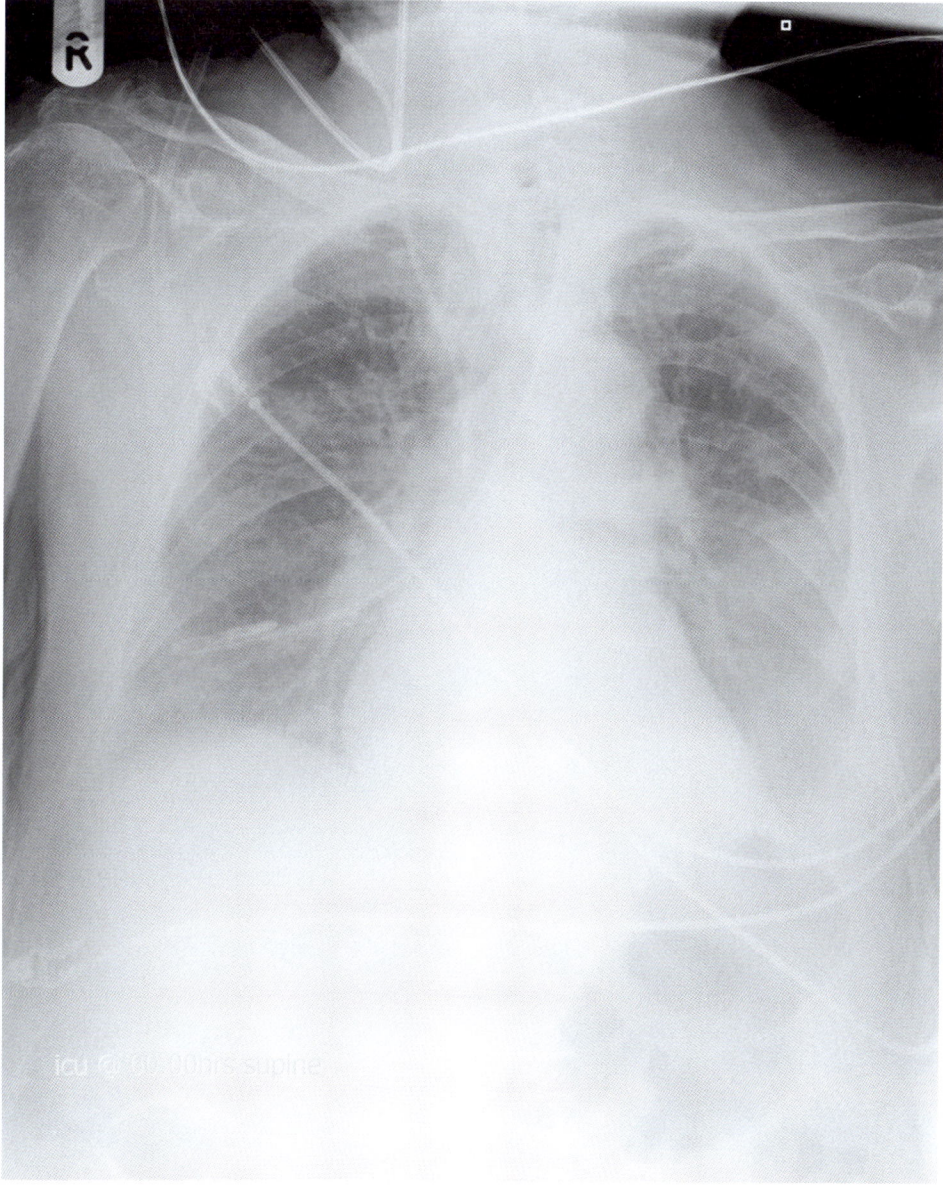

Figure 12.30

Answer to Case 14

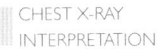

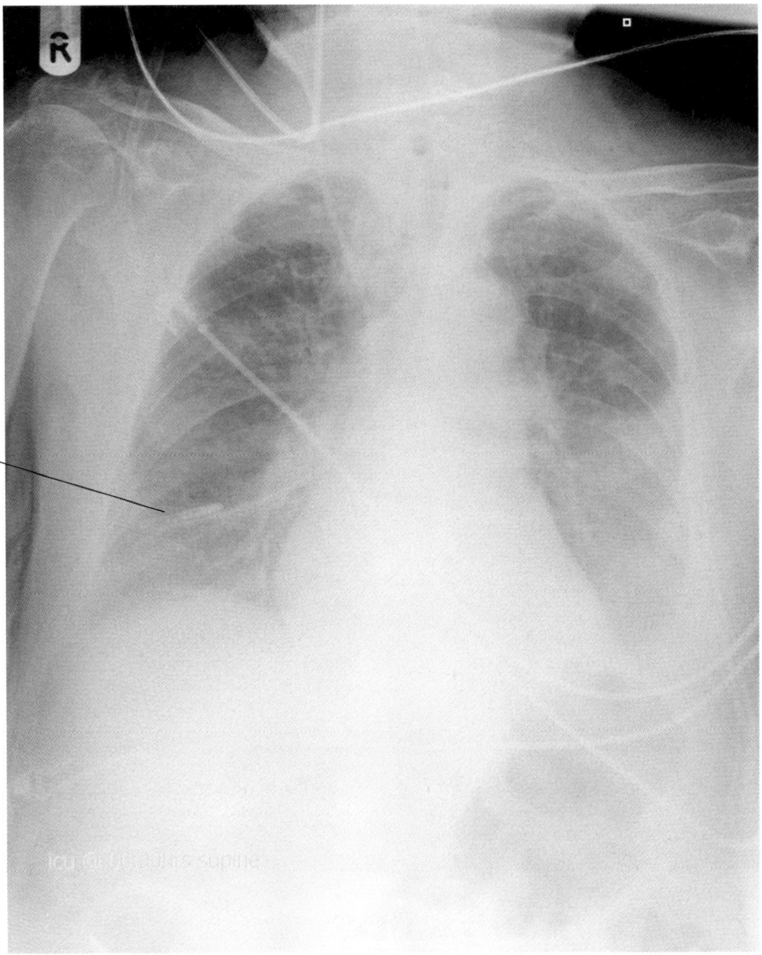

Figure 12.31

The NG tube is in the right bronchus intermedius and beyond. It is unsafe to feed the patient and the tube needs to be removed immediately. Please see Chapter 9 for more detailed information on NG tube placement.

Case 15

What has happened, and why?

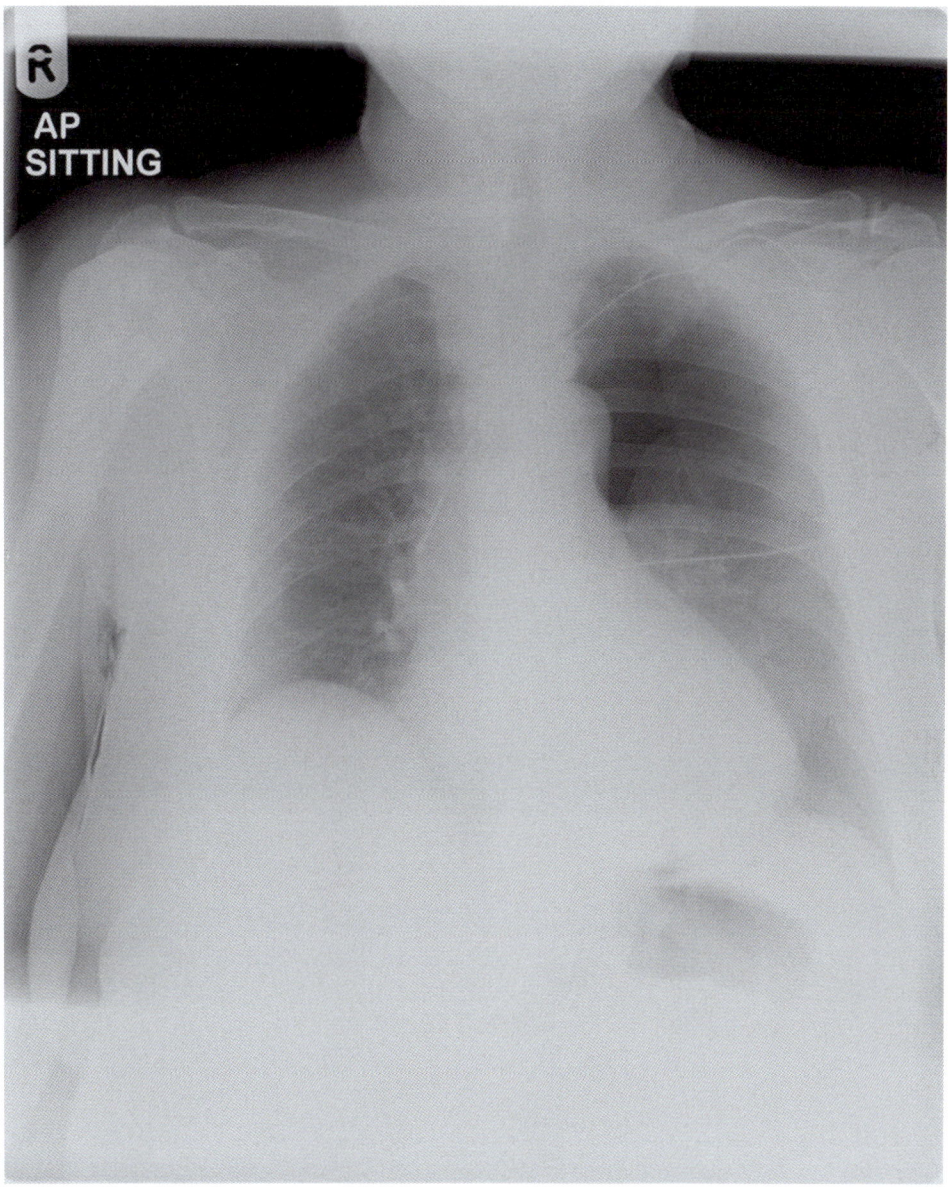

Figure 12.32

Answer to Case 15

There is a left-sided pneumothorax due to insertion of the left subclavian line. Please see Chapter 9 for more detailed information on placement of lines.

Case 16

Identify the device on the chest x-ray and comment on it.

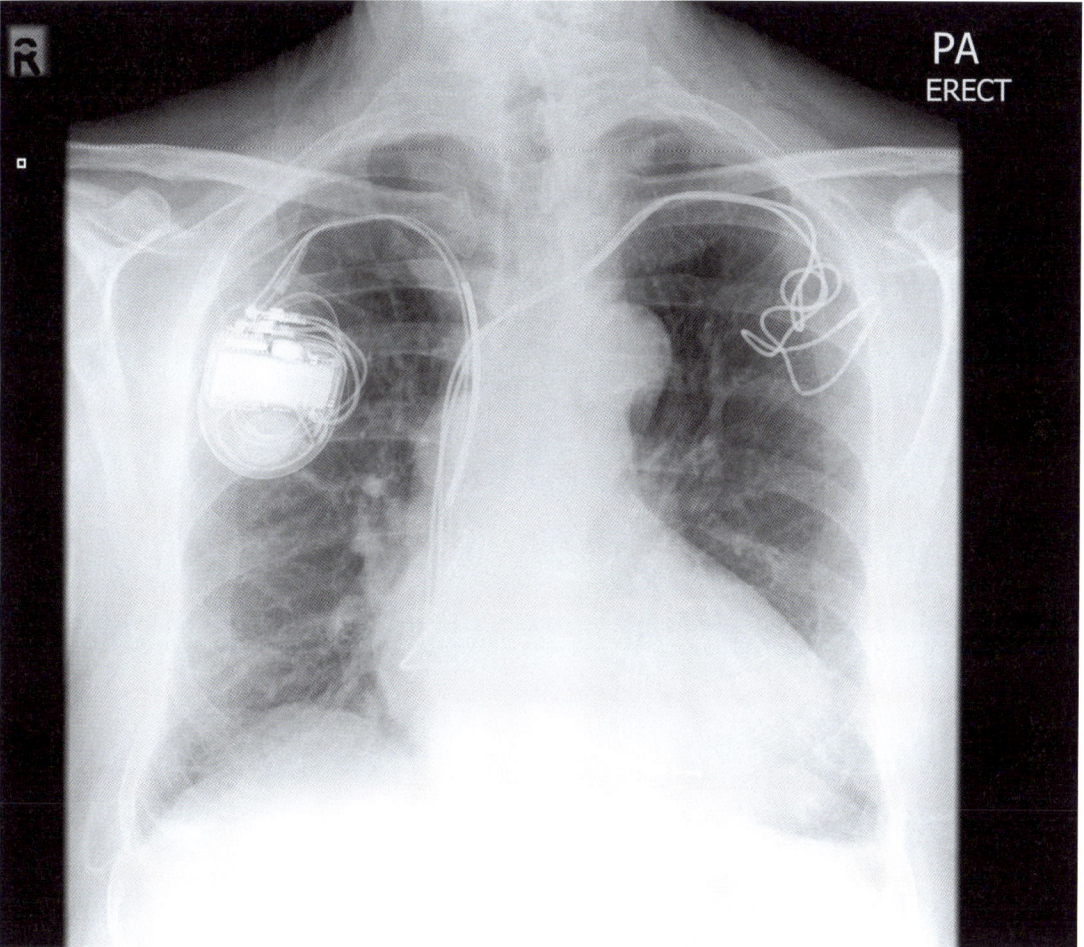

Figure 12.33

Answer to Case 16

There is a new automated implantable cardioverter defibrillator (AICD) on the right, and old wires remain on the left from a previous one. When replacing a pacemaker or AICD, it is quite common to leave the old wires in situ (as it is too difficult to remove them), and just remove the box.

The aim of an AICD is to stop abnormal rhythm (arrhythmia) with a burst of high-speed pacing (cardioversion). If this does not work, it acts as a defibrillator, giving an electric shock to restart the heart. The device also collects and stores information about the heart's electrical impulses. On the chest image, an AICD looks very similar to a pacemaker, except that you can see a thickened area along one of the wires; this is the difference in appearance.

Case 17

Comment on this image.

How would you confirm your suspicions?

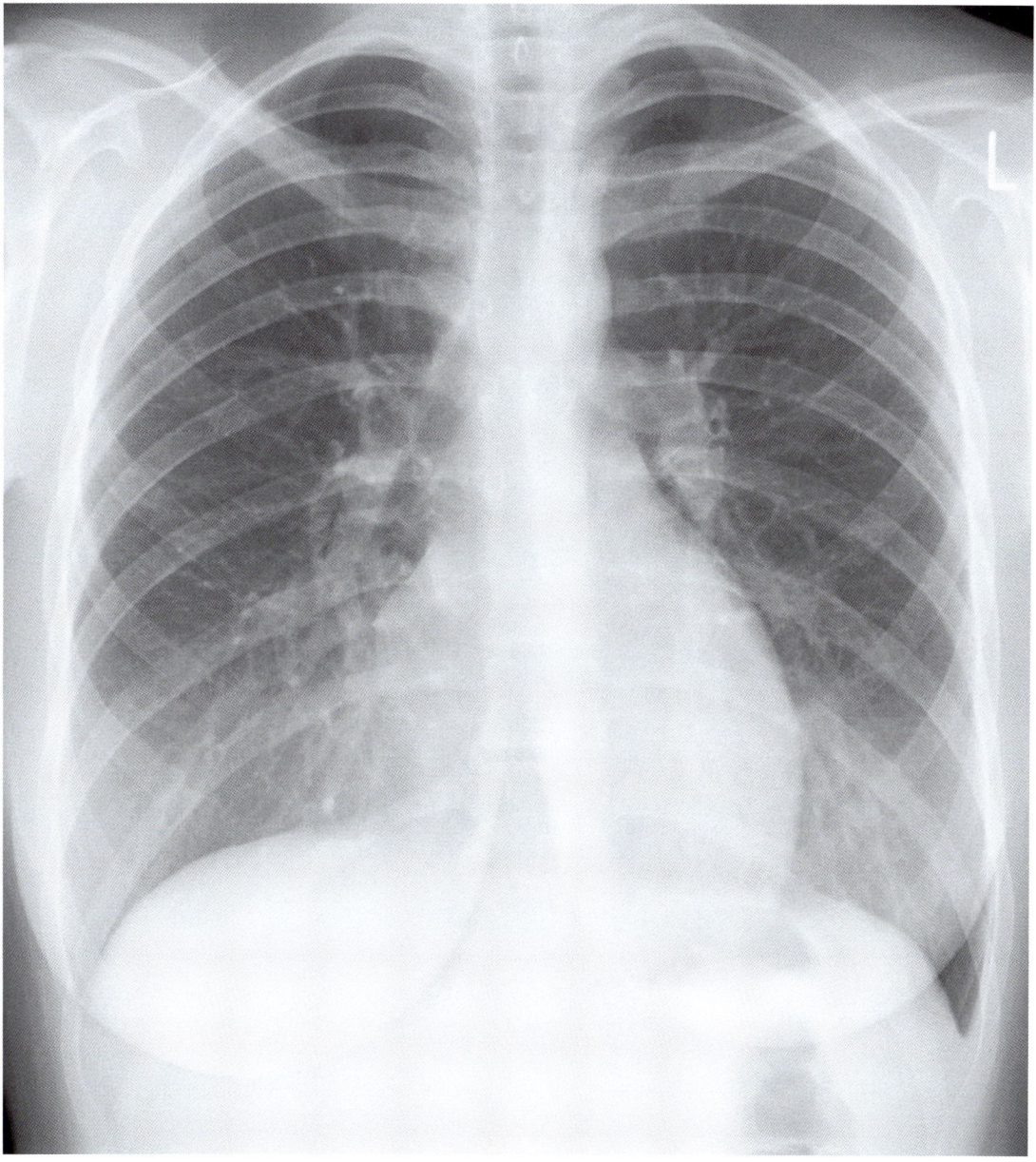

Figure 12.34

Answer to Case 17

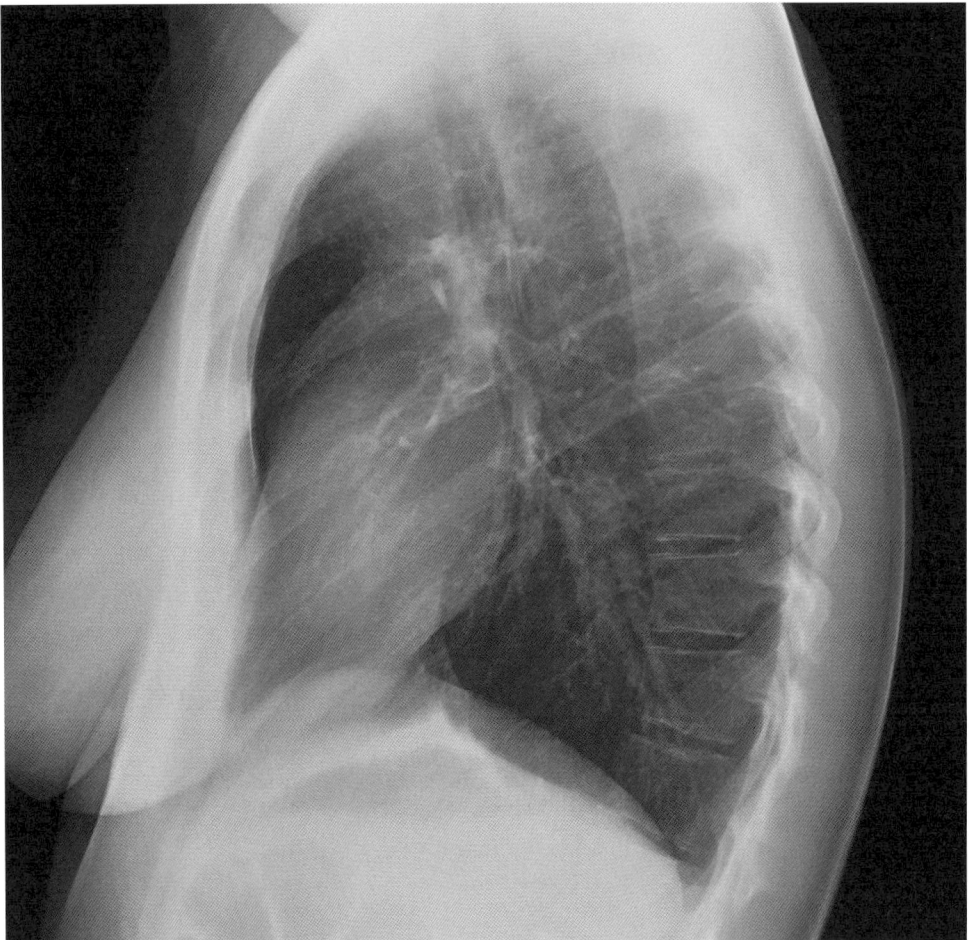

Figure 12.35

This image demonstrates pectus excavatum. The ribs on the right side are more parallel than those on the left, and the right heart border is slightly ill defined (not to be confused with consolidation). The best way to confirm this is to ask the radiographer who took the image whether they noticed if the anterior chest wall appeared slightly concave. Another option is to look and see if a lateral chest x-ray has been taken previously. This patient had a lateral chest image from a previous attendance, which confirmed it.

Case 18

Clinical details: increasing shortness of breath.

Comment on the image.

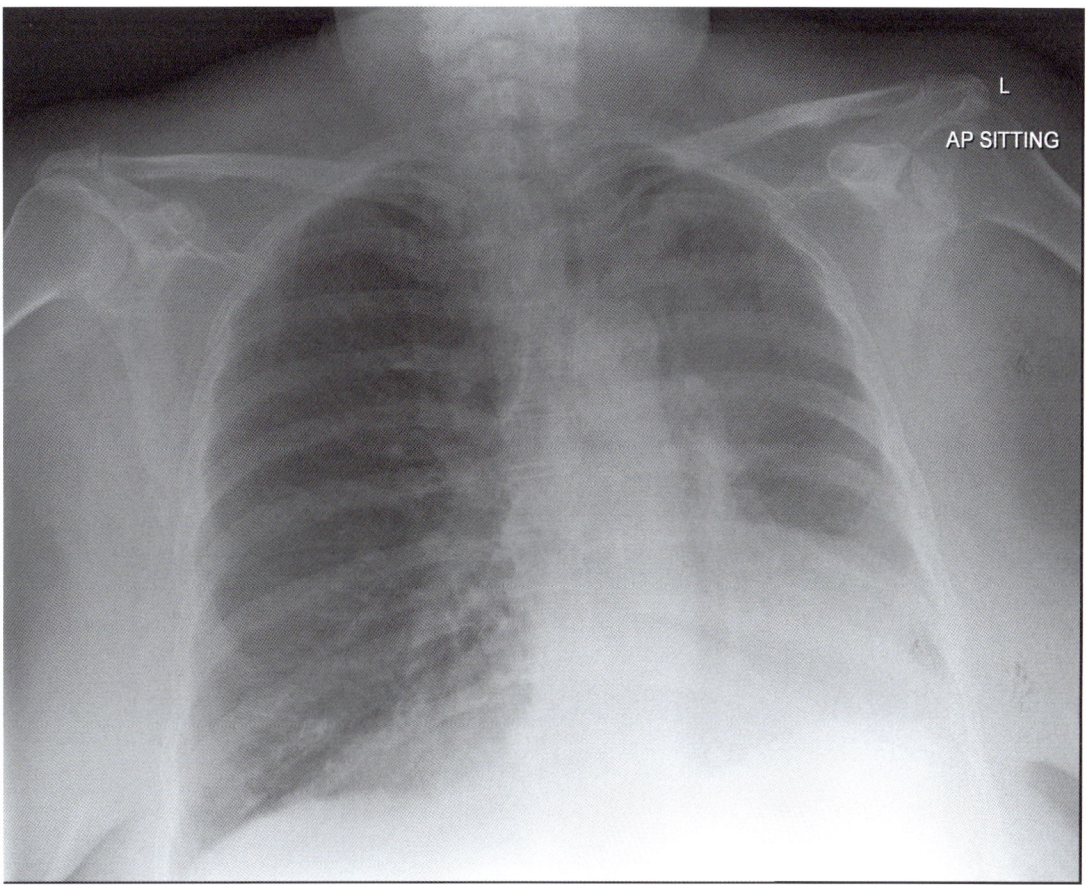

Figure 12.36

Answer to Case 18

There is left upper lobe collapse, demonstrated by loss of the clear definition of the left upper mediastinum/heart shadow, and a veil-like appearance on the left lung. Notice how the upper mediastinum is beginning to be pulled towards the collapsed side to take up the space caused by the collapsed lung.

This may be caused by a mucous plug, or a mass blocking off the airway. Further investigation with HRCT is required. In this case it was a carcinoid that caused the collapse of the lung.

Case 19

Clinical details: elderly patient fell onto right side, pain in chest. No other images taken.

Comment on the image.

What would you suggest happens next?

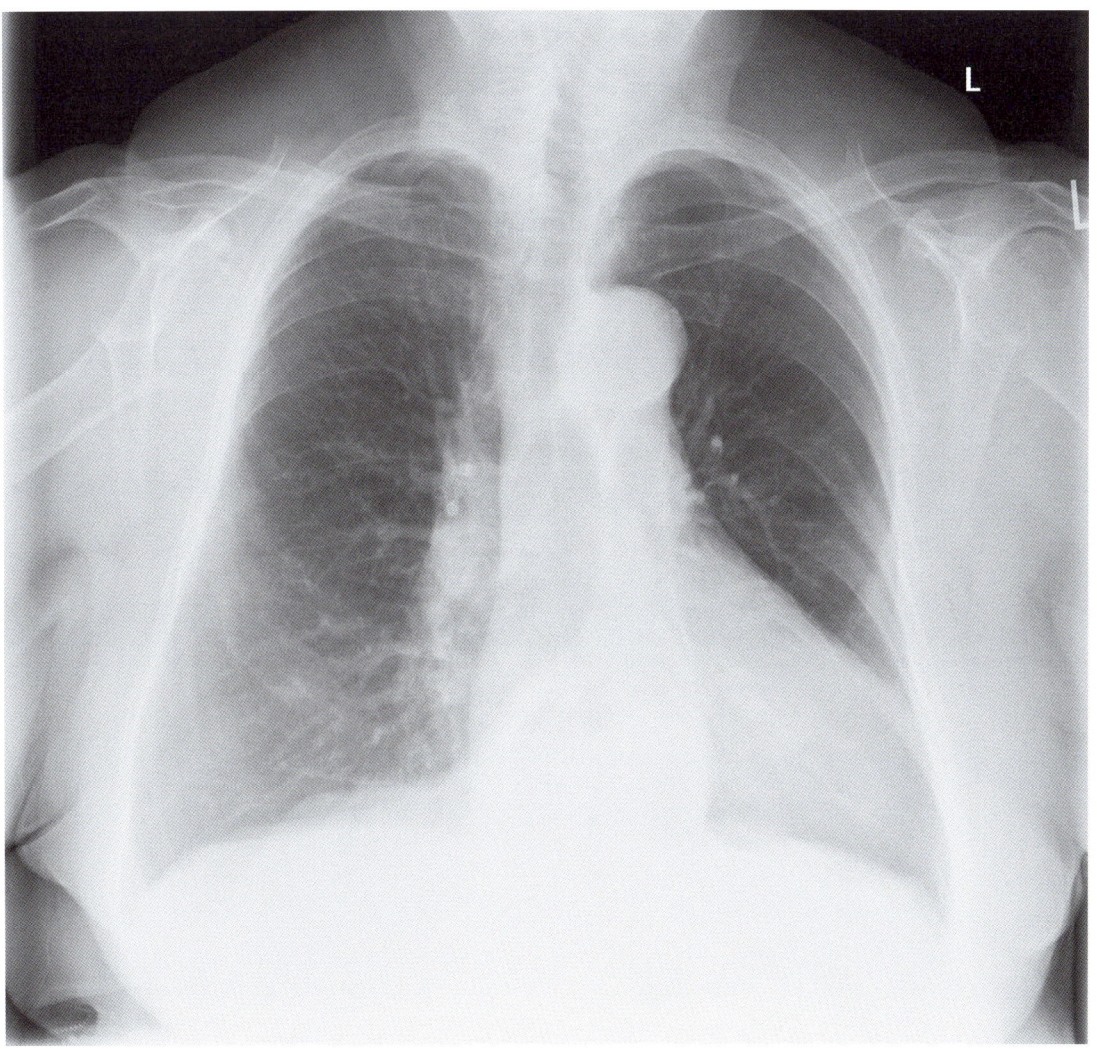

Figure 12.37

Answer to Case 19

There is anterior dislocation of the right humeral head as a result of the fall. No further bony injury is demonstrated. There is no sign of a chest infection or lung collapse, which may have resulted in the patient's fall.

Dedicated right shoulder images need to be done and the patient should be taken straight to A&E for her shoulder dislocation to be reduced.

This demonstrates that one should look at everything on the radiographic image, especially at the edges of the image, no matter what the image is of.

A large heart is noted, but no other signs of heart failure. A hiatus hernia is also noted.

Case 20

Clinical details: query chest infection?

Comment on the image.

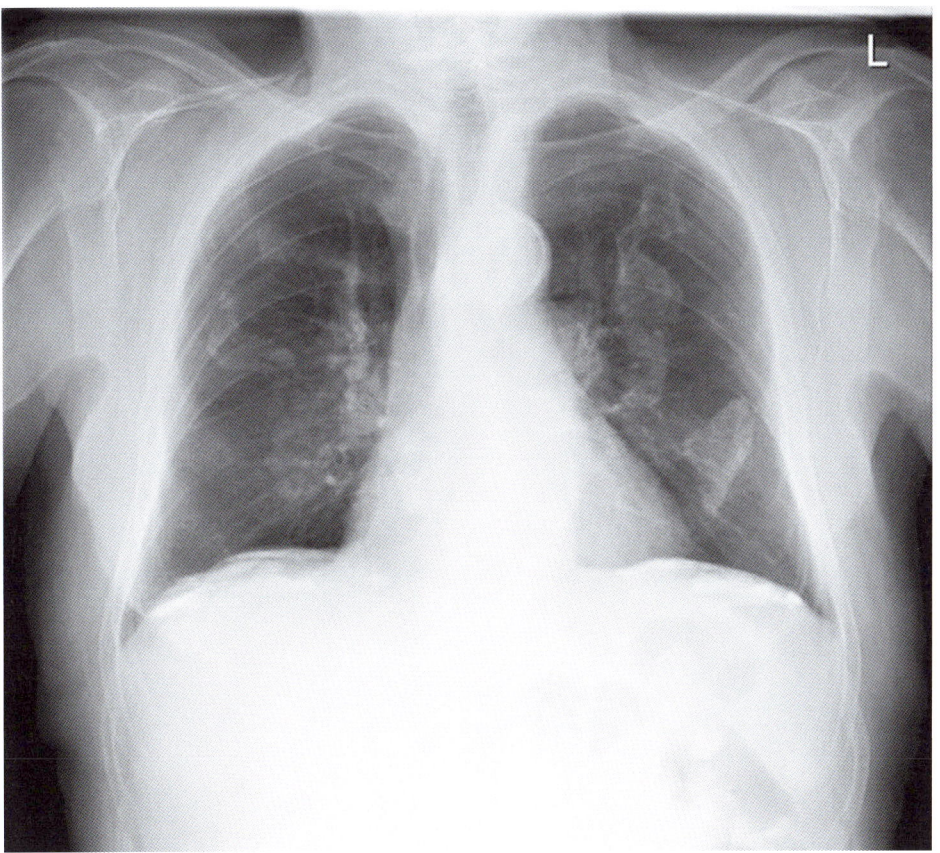

Figure 12.38

Answer to Case 20

There is no sign of consolidation or collapse on this radiograph. However, there are multiple pleural plaques due to previous asbestos exposure. These are classically demonstrated along both hemidiaphragms, but also elsewhere. Asbestos fibres travel to the periphery of the lung, perforate the visceral pleura and set up an inflammatory reaction, as visceral and parietal pleura rub together during respiration. This results in pleural plaques on the hemidiaphragms and laterally as they follow the contours of the ribs.

An old fracture of the left 6th posterior rib is also noted.

Case 21

Clinical details: increased shortness of breath. Query pneumothorax?

Is there a pneumothorax?

What normal variant can be identified?

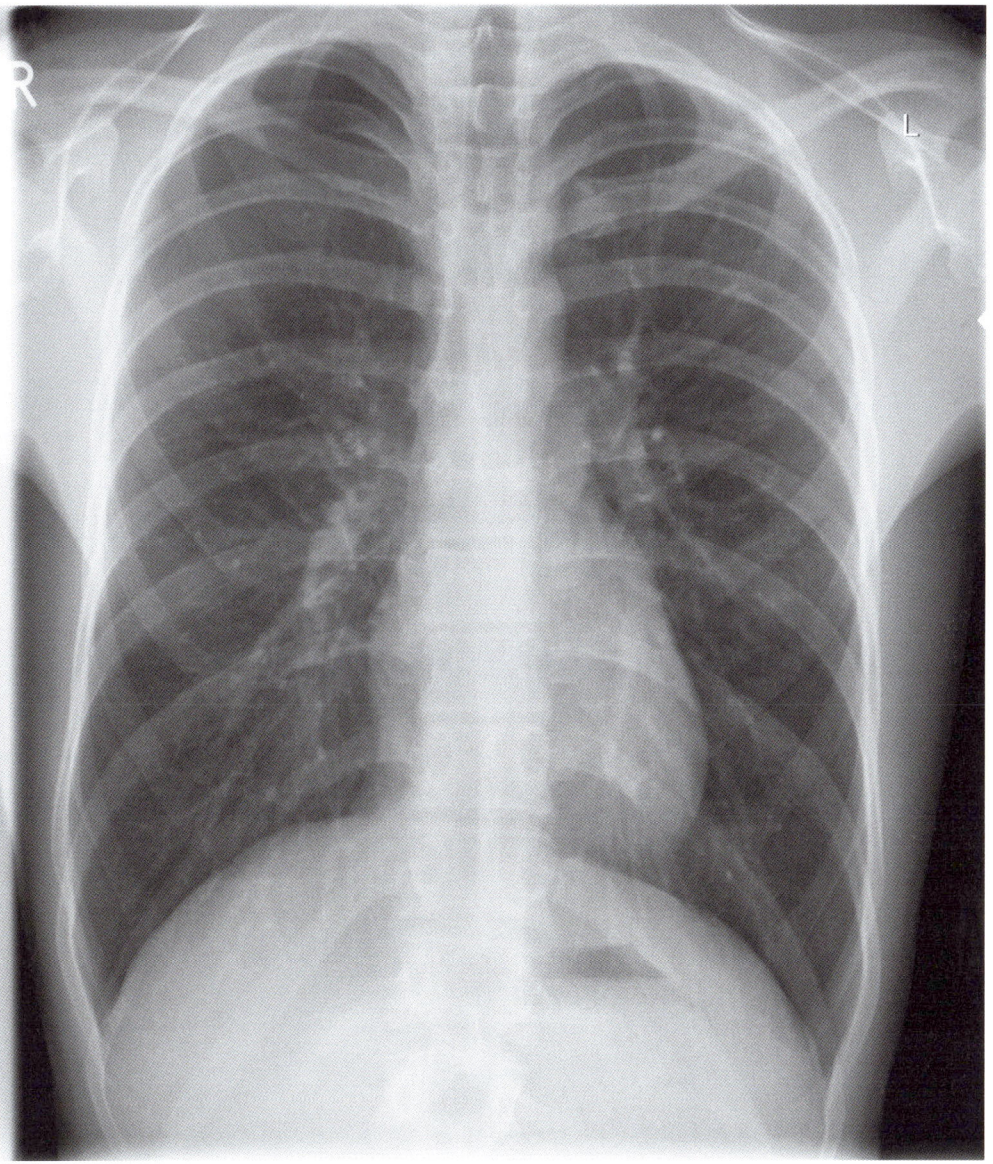

Figure 12.39

Answer to Case 21

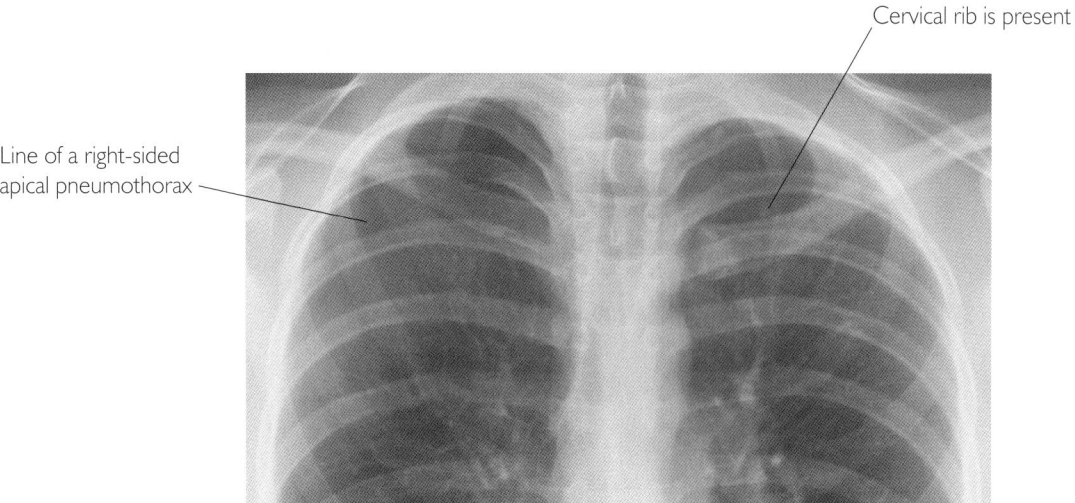

Figure 12.40

There is a subtle right apical pneumothorax. (This is where magnification and windowing are useful.) Also demonstrated are cervical ribs, which should be mentioned in the report. Even though they may not be causing any problem at the time of imaging, they may do in the future.

Case 22

Clinical details: patient on intensive care, being ventilated.

Query pneumothorax?

Comment on the image.

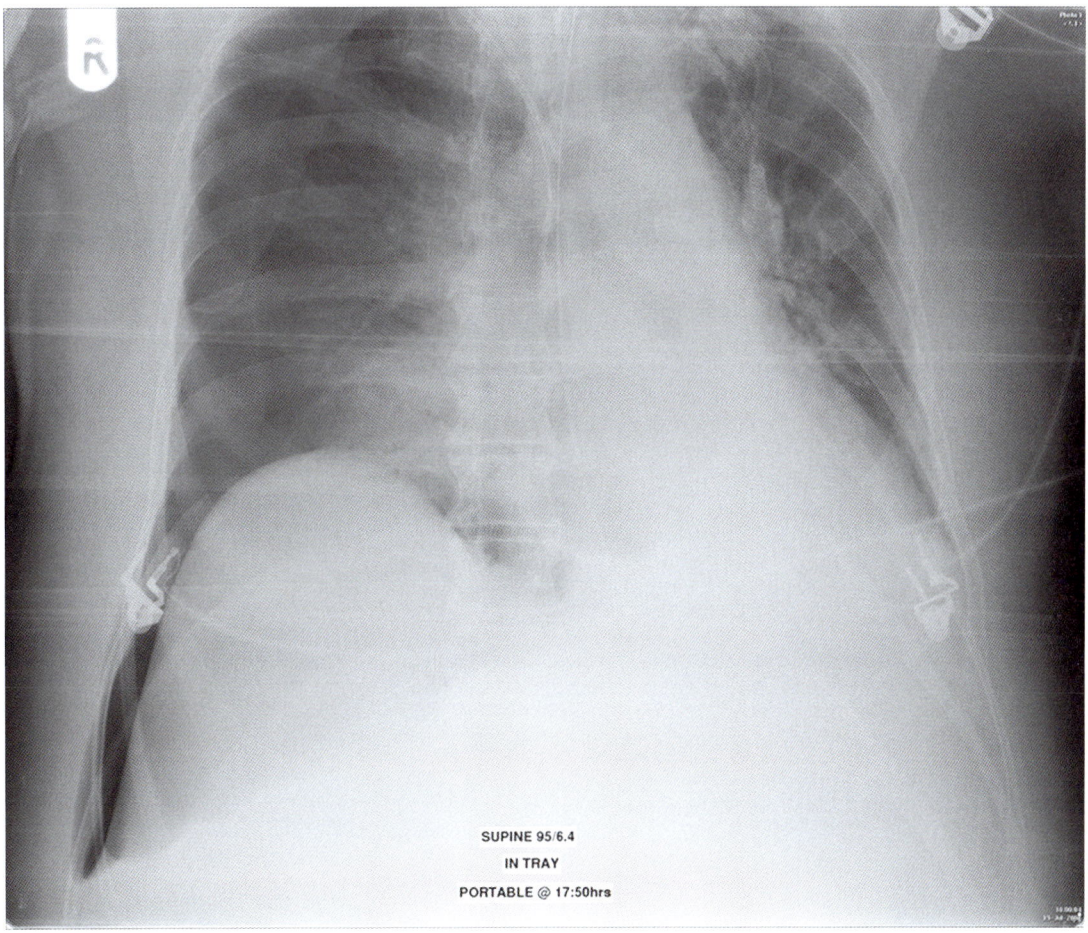

Figure 12.41

Answer to Case 22

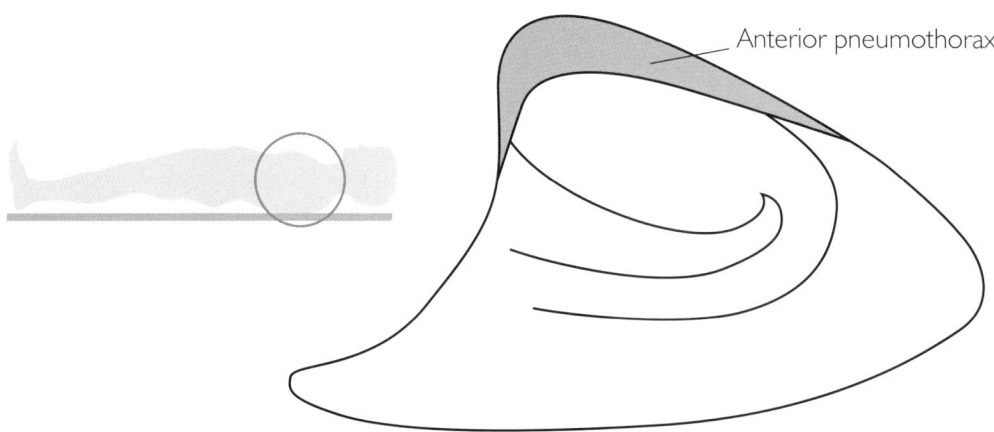

Figure 12.42
Lungs in a supine patient; air will rise, whereas fluid (effusion) will settle posteriorly

There is air with no lung markings above and lateral to the right diaphragm, making a sharp contrast with the right diaphragm. This is the deep sulcus sign of a pneumothorax in a supine patient; also noted is movement of the heart and mediastinum away from the right-sided pneumothorax. A small pneumothorax in a ventilated patient can quickly become serious, resulting in a tension pneumothorax.

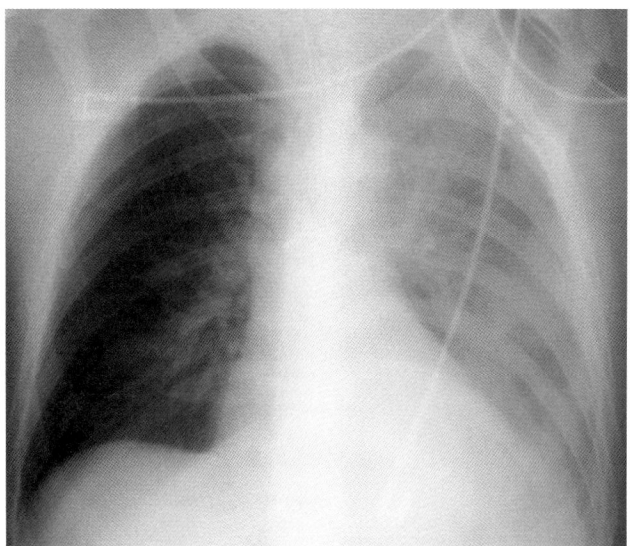

Figure 12.43 Left-sided effusion in a supine patient

Case 23

Clinical details: inpatient being nursed supine, sudden increase in breathing difficulties. Query pneumothorax, lung collapse or consolidation?

Comment on the image.

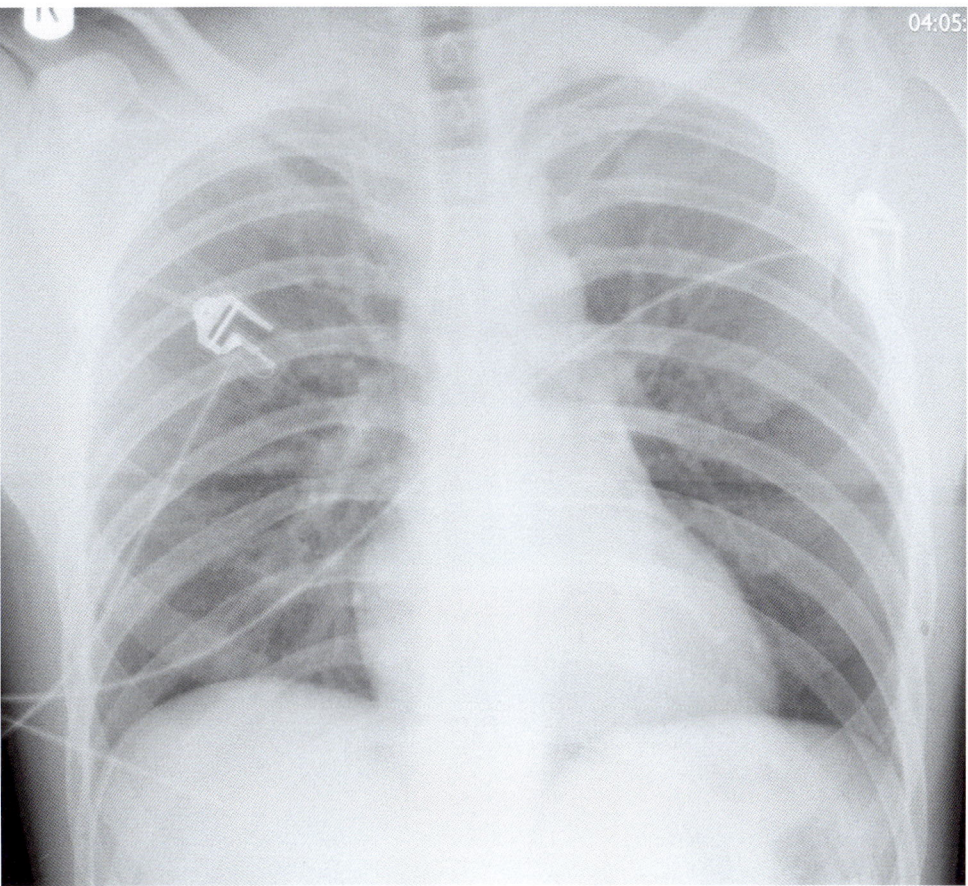

Figure 12.44

Answer to Case 23

The area above the left diaphragm and behind the heart is more lucent than normal, and to a lesser extent is also lucent above the right diaphragm, although subtler. Remember this is a supine patient. This is the deep sulcus sign of a pneumothorax in a supine patient, a very subtle sign in this patient.

Compare to the previous case.

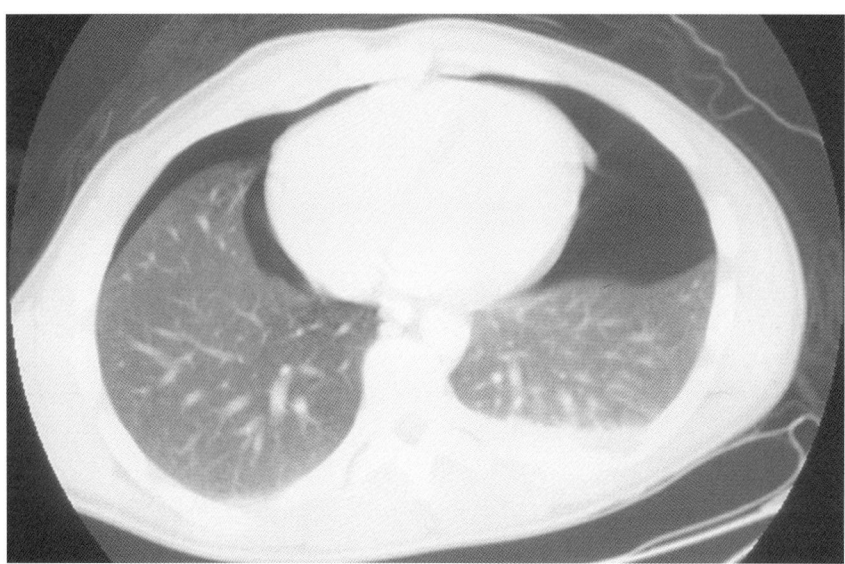

Figure 12.45

A CT scan was done to confirm the diagnosis.

The CT confirms that what was only a subtle finding on the chest image, is actually a large bilateral pneumothorax.

Case 24

Clinical details: evidence of chest infection which antibiotics have not cleared.

Query any remaining consolidation?

Comment on the image.

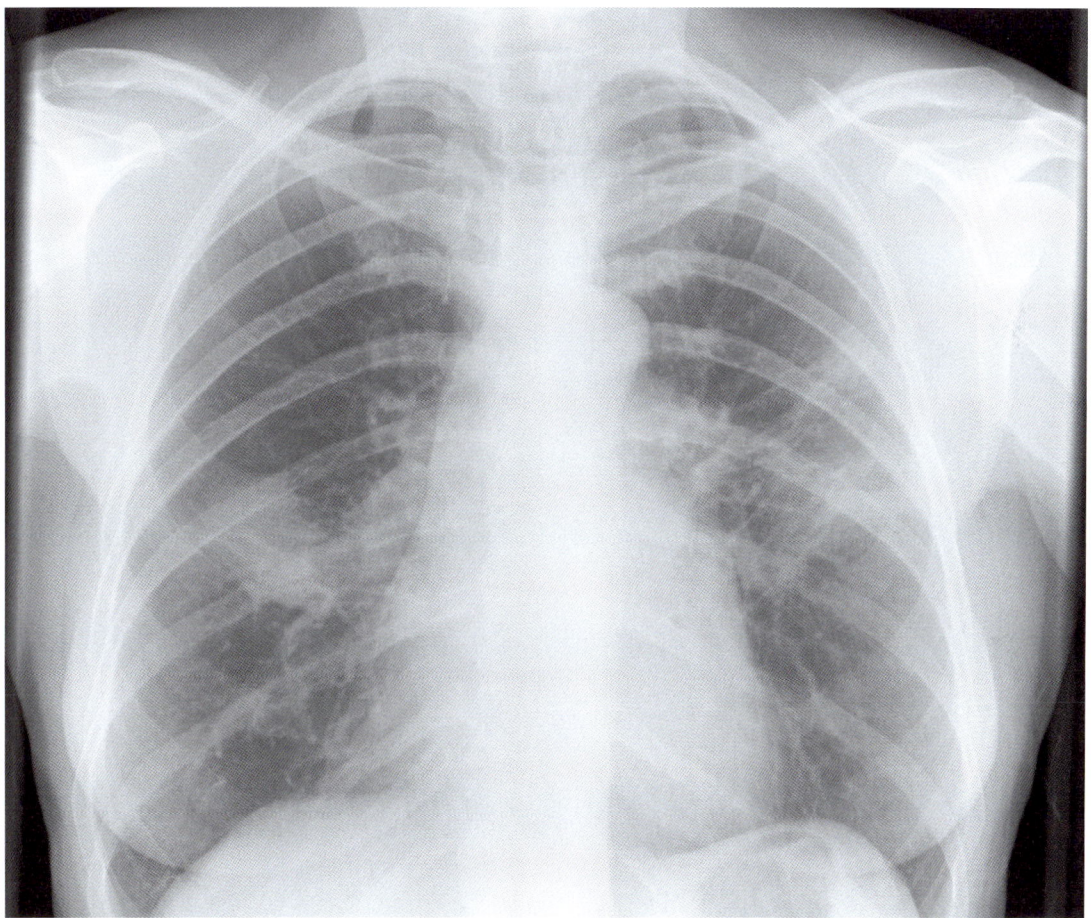

Figure 12.46

Answer to Case 24

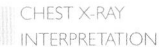

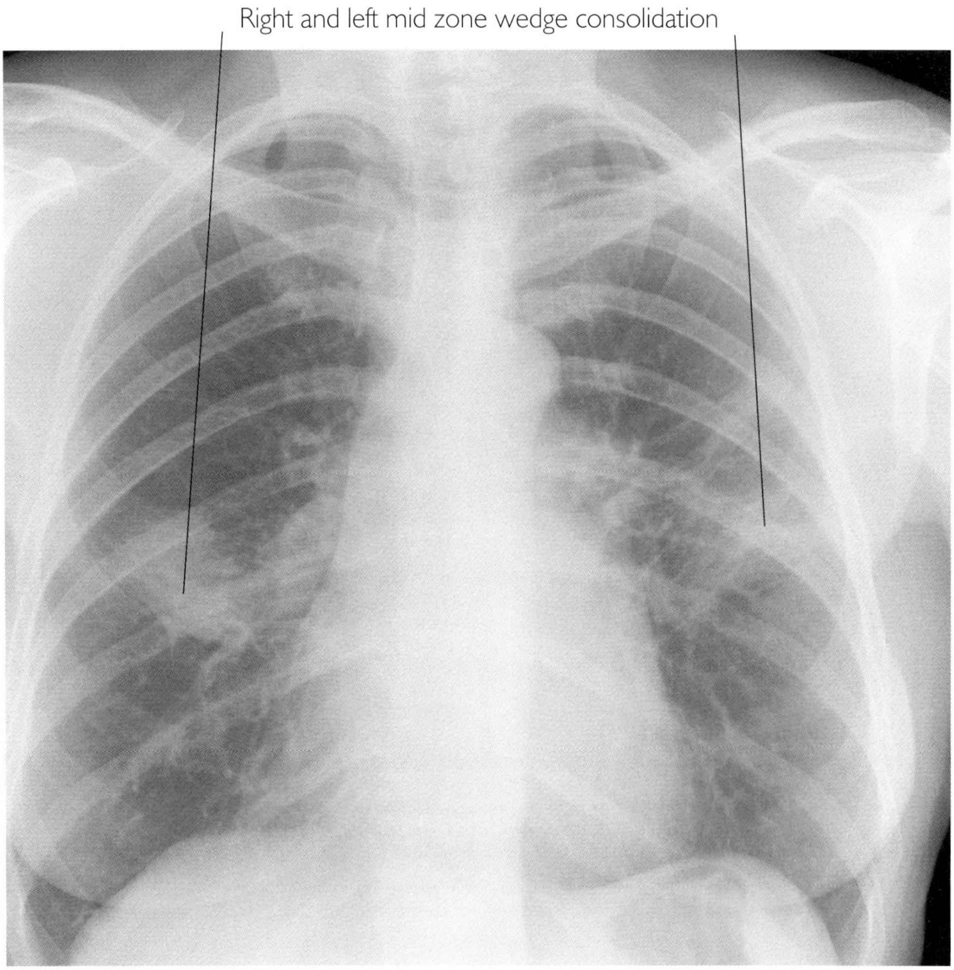

Figure 12.47

There is right and left mid zone wedge consolidation. Considering the clinical details, this is most likely the result of an infective process. Suggest continue to treat as infection, with repeat x-ray after 6–8 weeks to check that infection has been resolved. If the consolidation has not significantly cleared by the next chest image, further investigation with HRCT will be required to assess if the cause of the consolidation is an underlying lung tumour blocking the bronchi.

Case 25

Clinical details: Query any signs of heart failure?

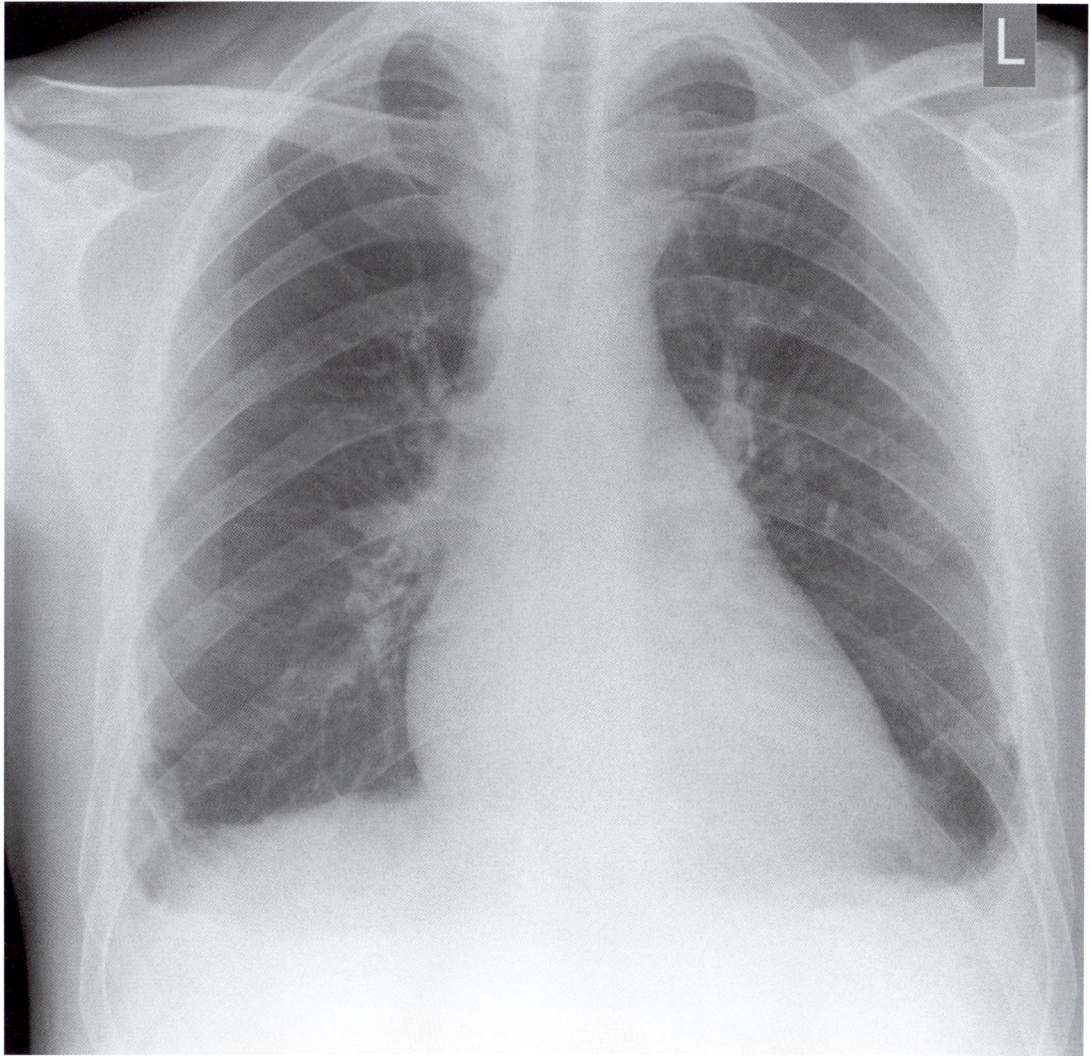

Figure 12.48

Answer to Case 25

There is an enlarged cardiothoracic ratio with small bilateral pleural effusions. No interstitial oedema demonstrated on this image. Appearance is consistent with heart failure. Suggest treat as heart failure, with repeat x-ray following treatment.

Case 26

Clinical details: routine chest x-ray following fracture neck of femur, prior to surgery. Comment on the image.

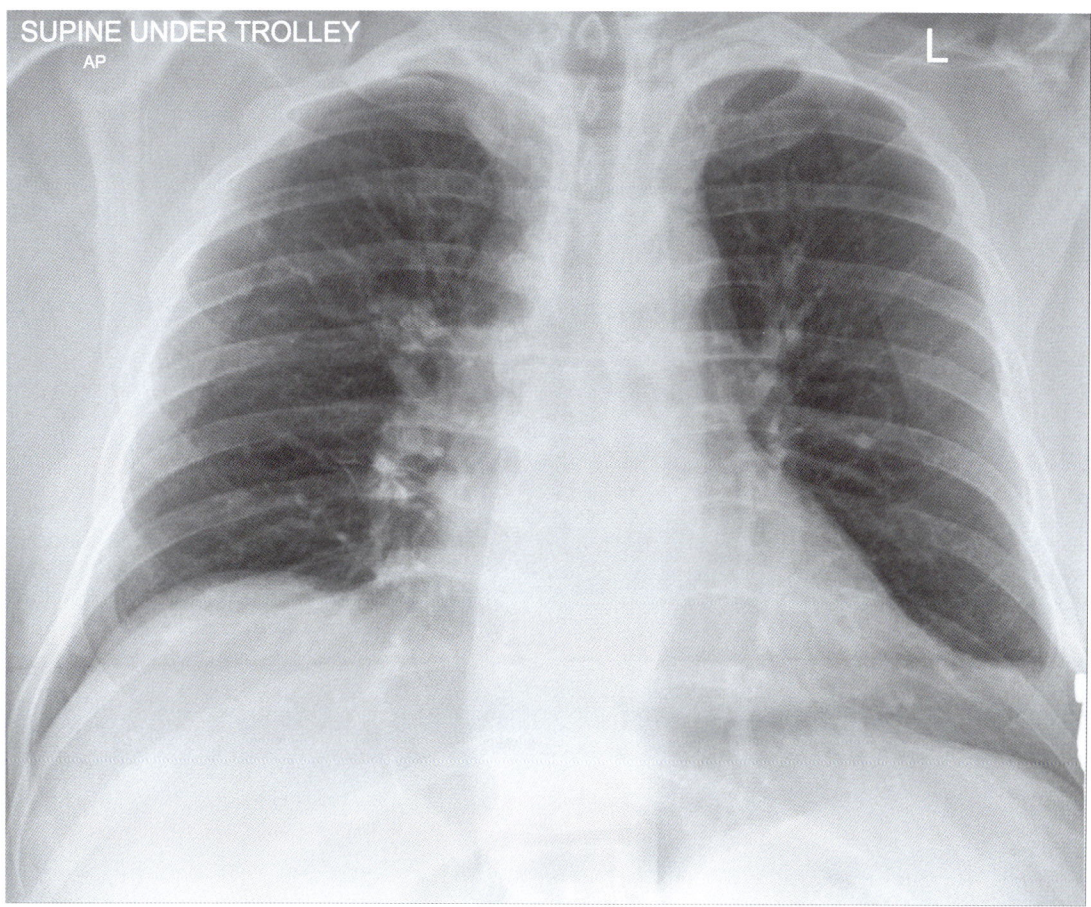

Figure 12.49

Answer to Case 26

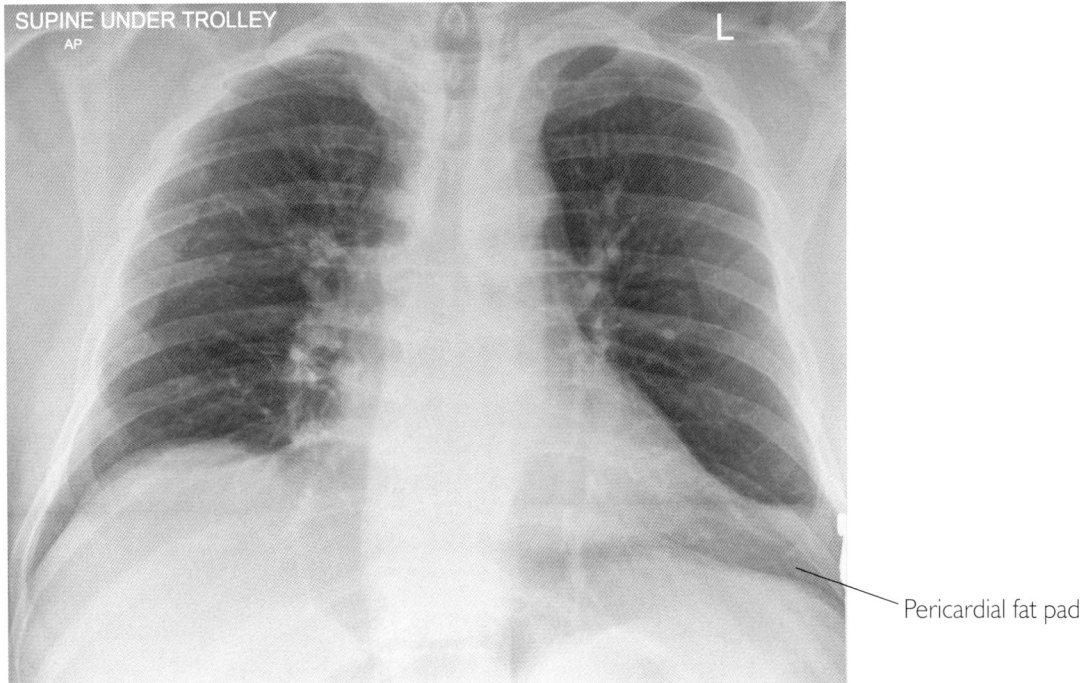

Figure 12.50

The patient is supine and, taking this into consideration, the heart size and mediastinum are within normal limits. There are no signs of heart failure, and no consolidation or collapse is demonstrated. However, there is a large left-sided pericardial fat pad. This should not be mistaken for collapsed lung or consolidation, although in some cases it can be difficult.

Case 27

Clinical details: has had difficulty breathing for a long while, now getting worse. Comment on the image.

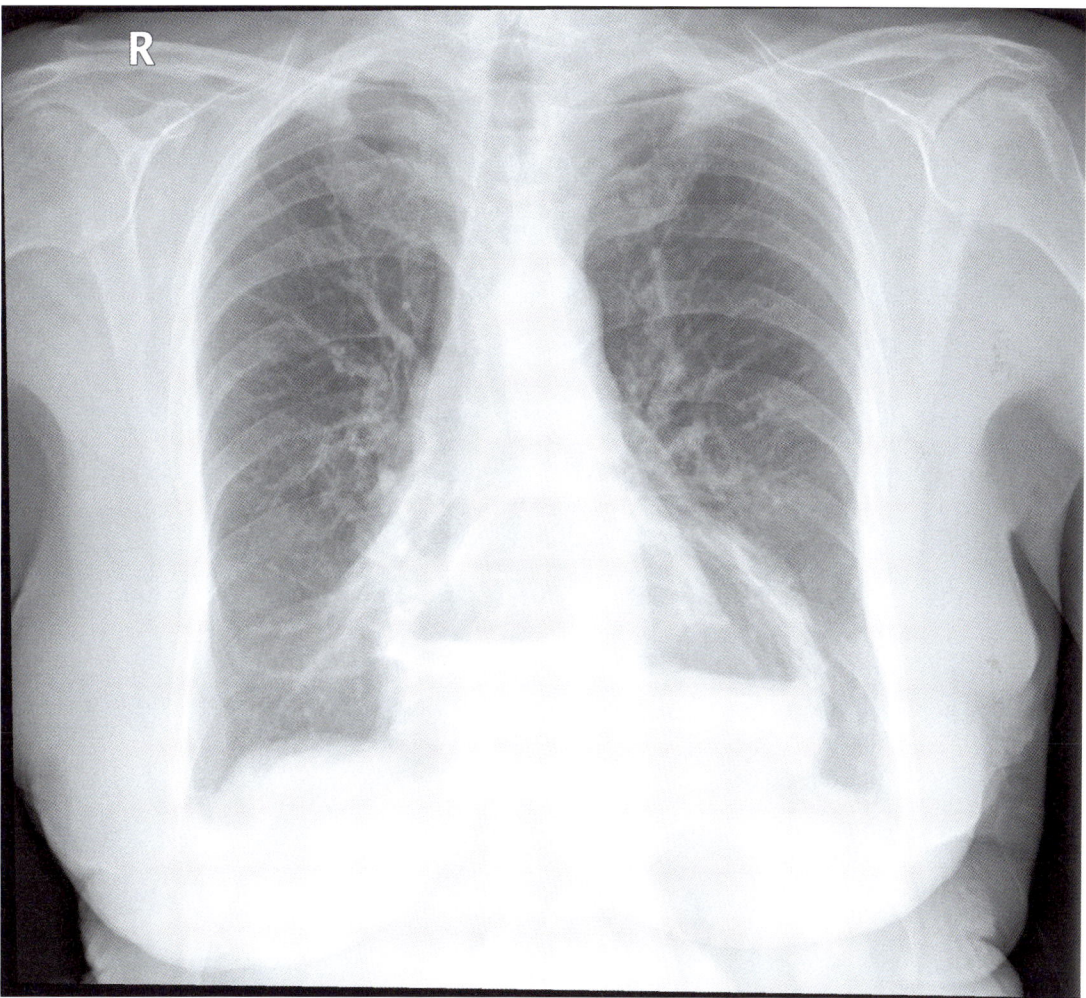

Figure 12.51

Answer to Case 27

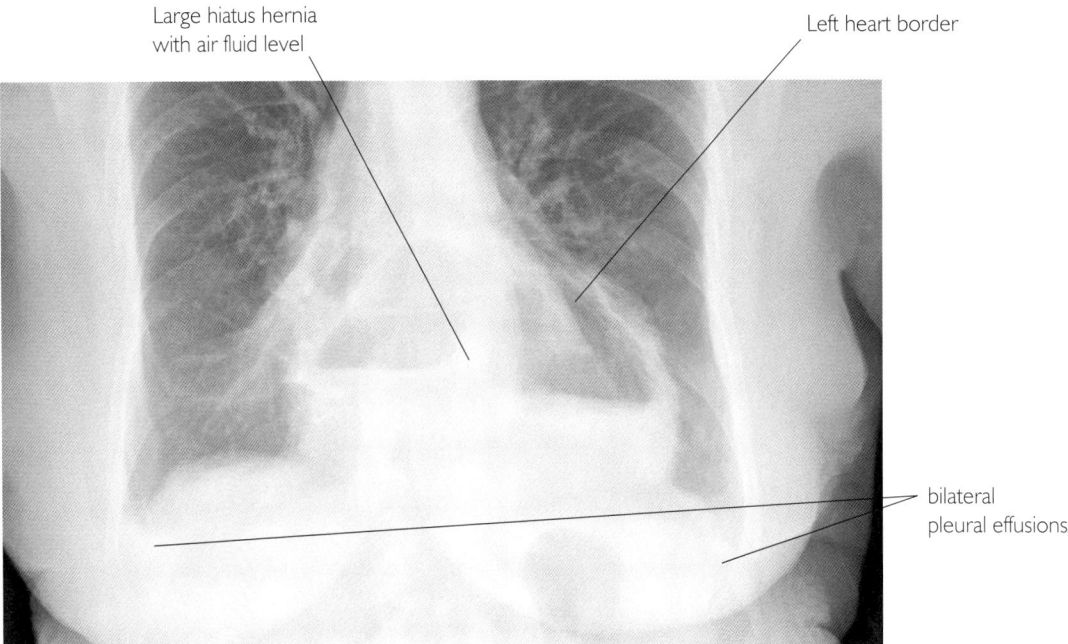

Figure 12.52

There is an extremely large hiatus hernia, which may explain why the patient has had long-term breathing difficulties. However, the heart does not appear enlarged. Small bilateral pleural effusions with suspicion of right sided Kerley Bs.

The x-ray appearances are consistent with heart failure, which would fit with the clinical details describing increased breathlessness.

Case 28

Clinical details: 50-year-old smoker, with ongoing cough and difficulty breathing. Comment on the image, and what should happen next.

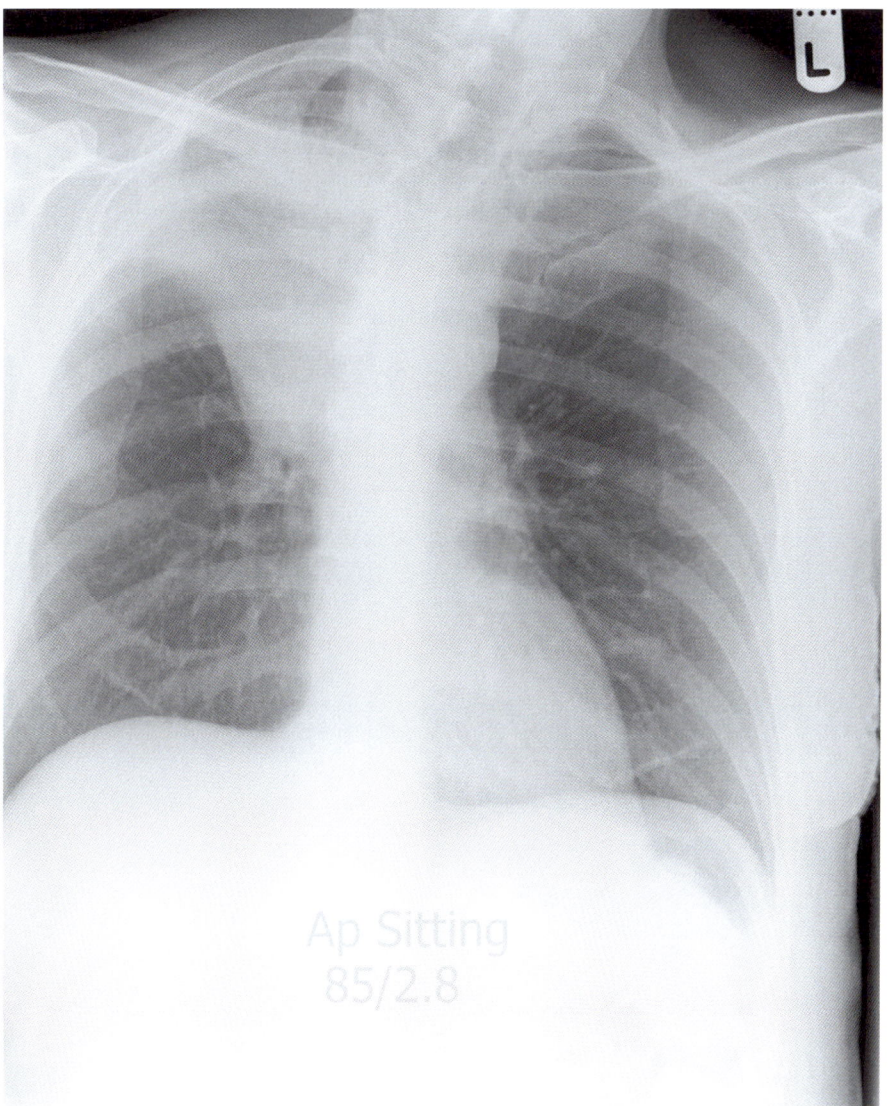

Figure 12.53

Answer to Case 28

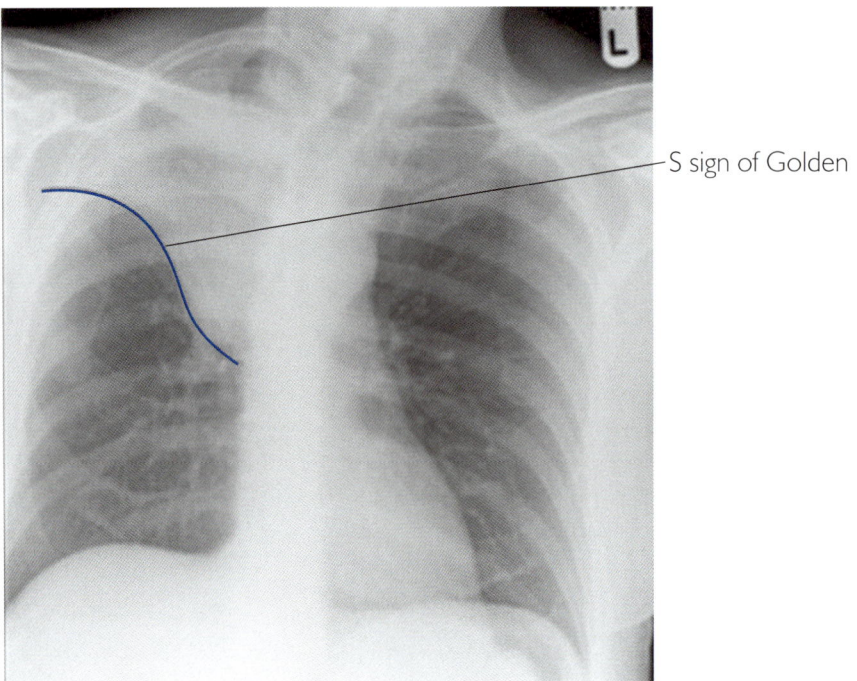

Figure 12.54

There is right upper lobe collapse, with a bulging of the right hilar. The collapse is caused by a lung tumour at the right hilar. In many texts, the line made by the right upper lobe collapse and hilar tumour is called the S sign of Golden – in other words it looks like the letter 'S'.

The patient requires a HRCT and referral to the lung cancer fast-track service.

Case 29

Comment on the image.

Before reviewing the lateral radiograph, can you work out (using Felson's silhouette sign) which part of the mediastinum the mass is in?

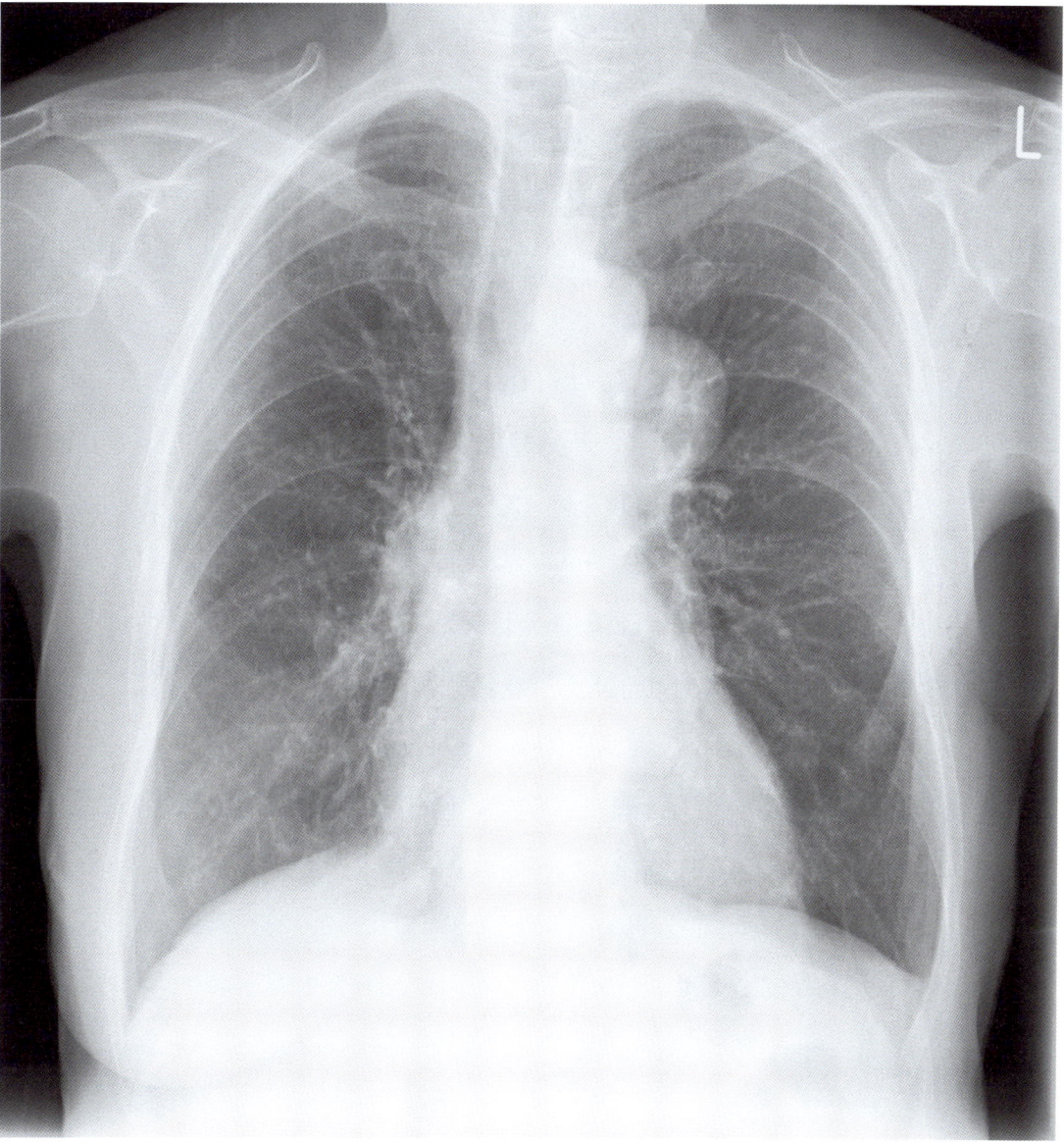

Figure 12.55

Answer to Case 29

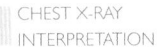

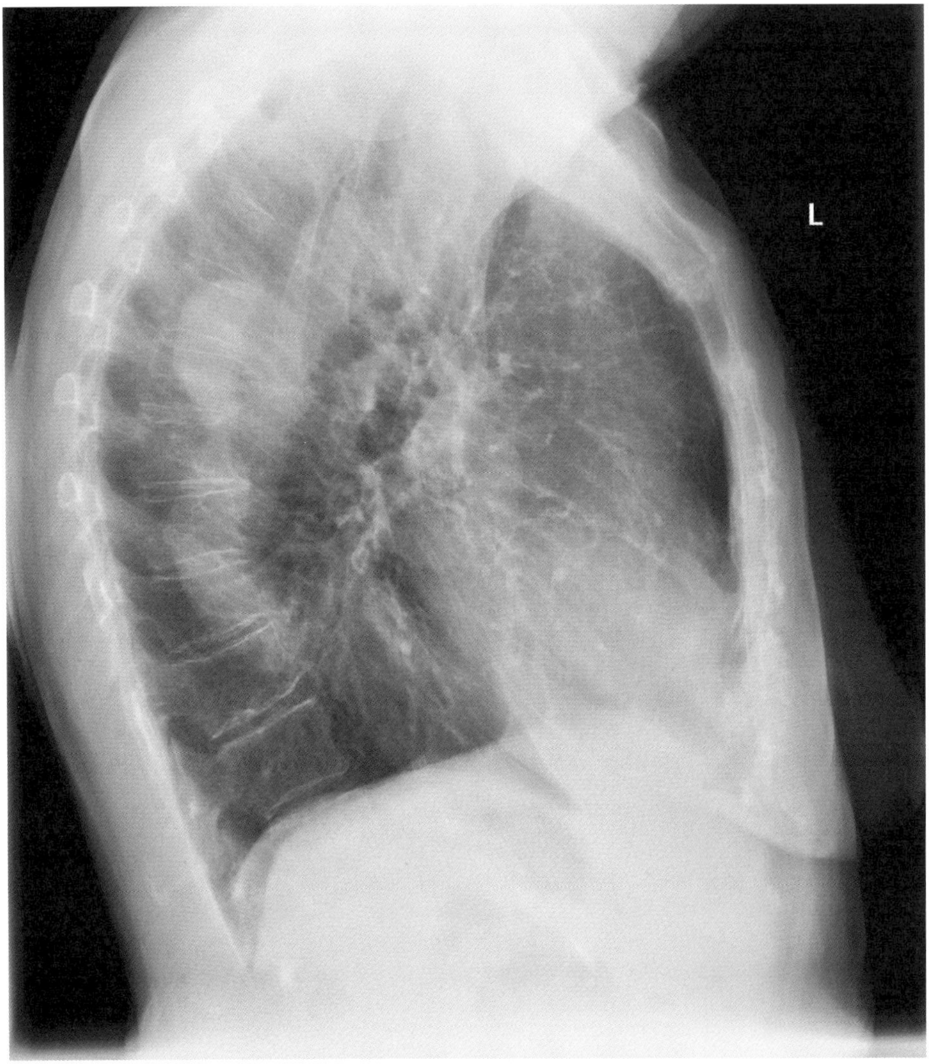

Figure 12.56

It is a posterior mediastinal mass, next to the aorta; it is an aortic aneurysm.

On the PA view, the lateral border of the heart and upper mediastinum could still be seen, even with the mass abutting it; hence, using Felson's silhouette sign, it is most likely a posterior mass.

Case 30

Clinical details: patient has known renal cancer. Query any metastases? Comment on the image.

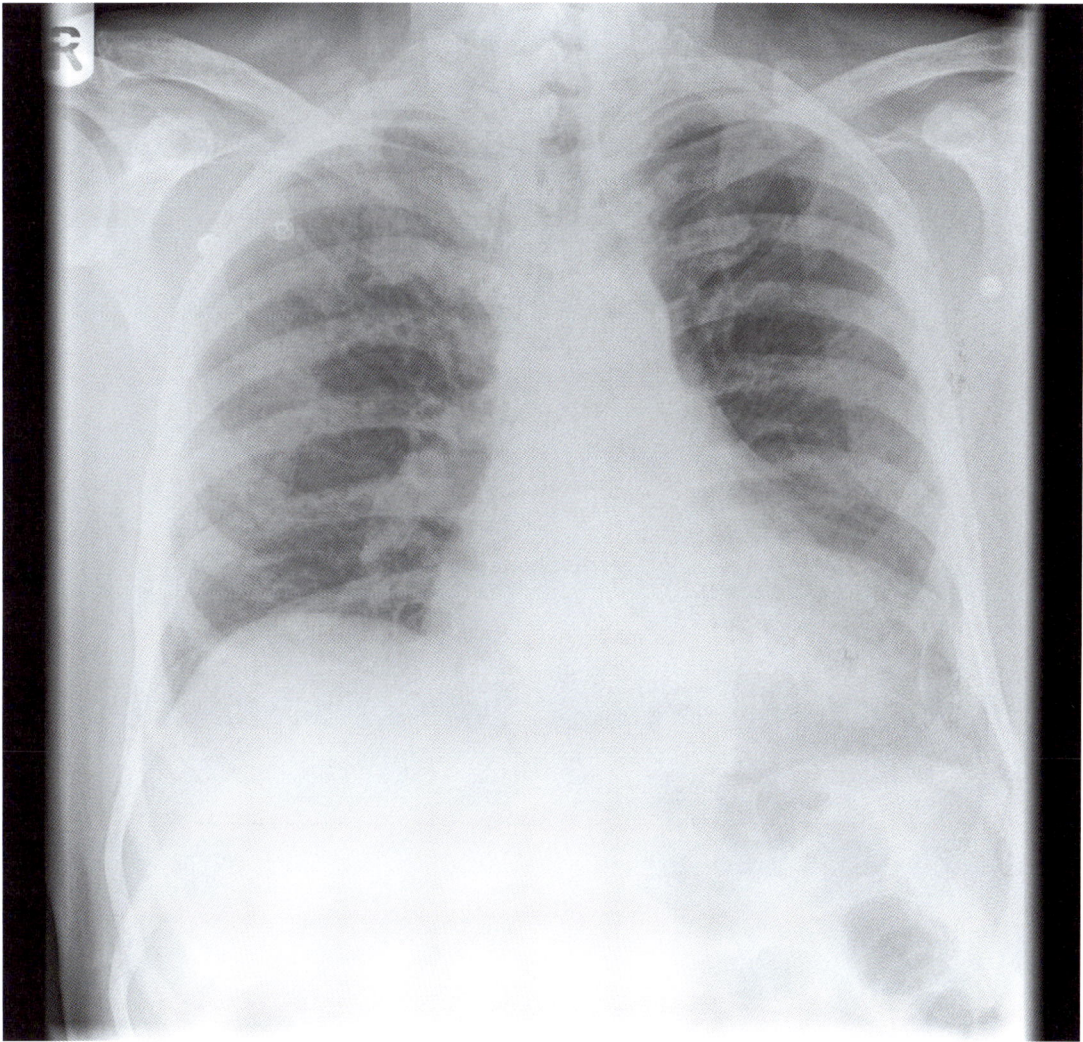

Figure 12.57

Answer to Case 30

If you look carefully at the density of the ribs, clavicle and part of the scapula, they are very sclerotic. This is a result of metastases. There are multiple metastases of the ribs, clavicle and scapula and this was confirmed on nuclear medicine scan.

Case 31

Clinical details: ongoing back pain, query chest related?

Comment on the images.

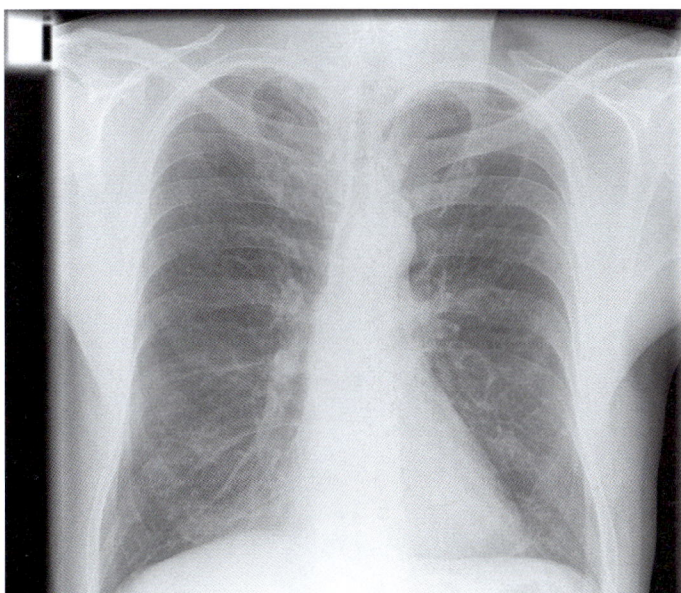

Figure 12.58

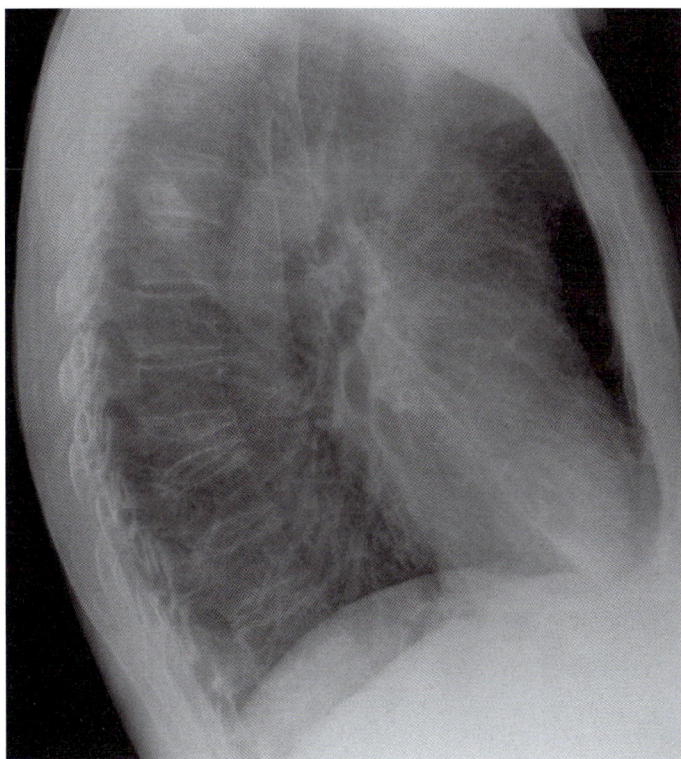

Figure 12.59

Answer to Case 31

The lateral view only demonstrated an increased rounded density over the upper thoracic spine. This did look suspicious for lung mass; hence a HRCT was done. This demonstrated that an unusually large osteophyte of the thoracic spine was causing the increased density, which explained why the patient had backache.

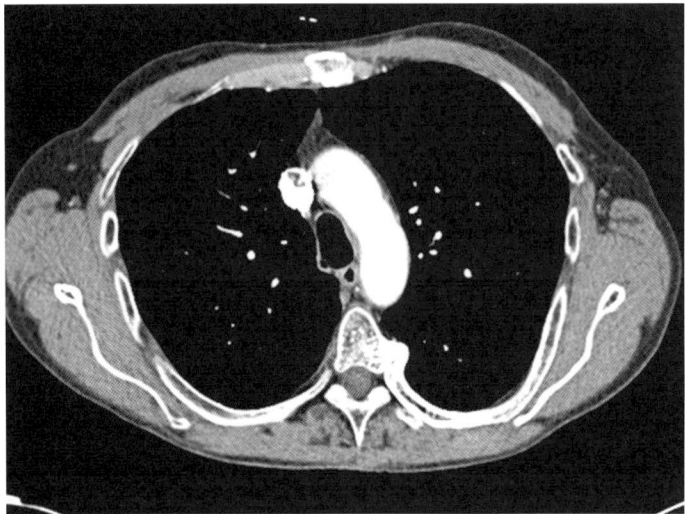

Figure 12.60

Case 32

Clinical details: 25-year-old immigrant lived in UK for 2 years. Cough for 2 months, starting to feel unwell. Query chest infection?

Comment on the image.

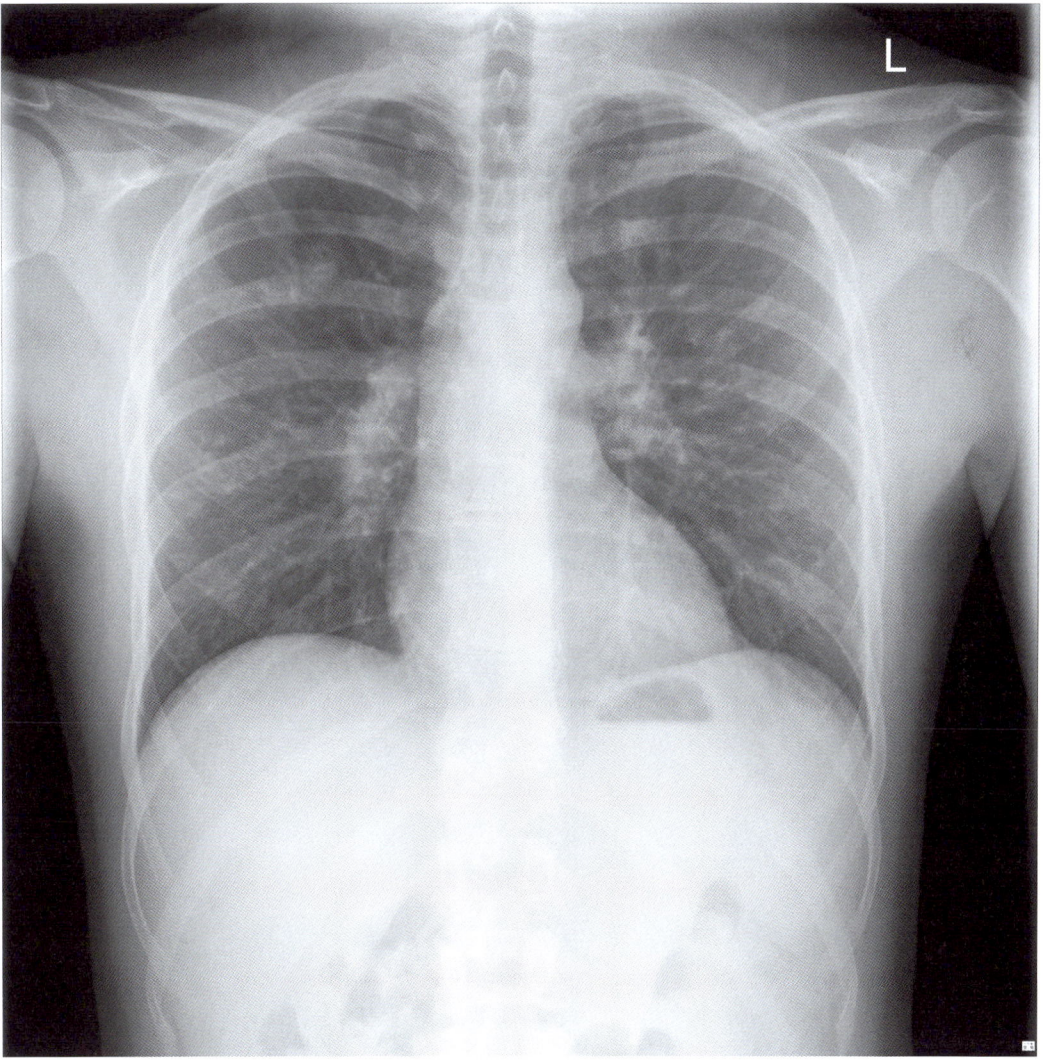

Figure 12.61

Answer to Case 32

There is patchy consolidation of the left lung, consistent with consolidation from an infective process. However, there is also a round air-filled opacity in the right upper zone, with a lobulated cystic type appearance. The patient was treated with antibiotics for the infection, with a repeat x-ray 8 weeks later. Both the hilar are bulky on this initial image which may be due to the infective process, but is also common in TB.

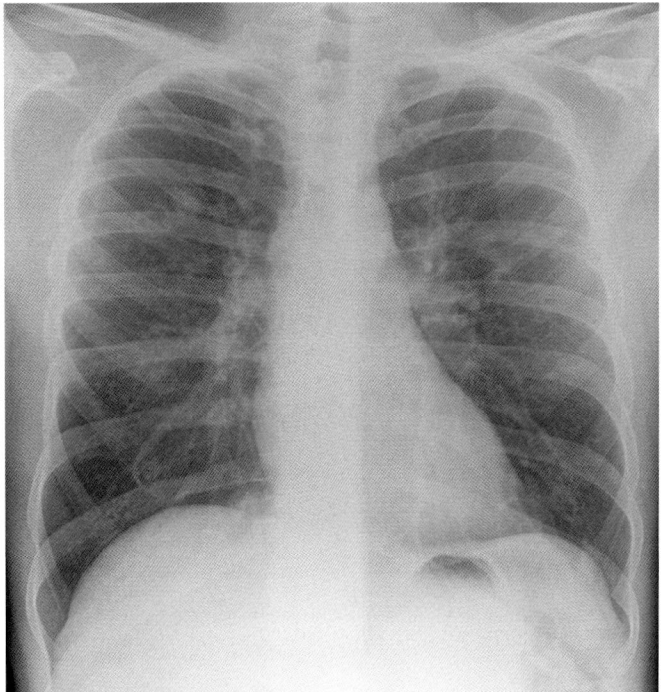

This repeat demonstrated that the left lung consolidation had cleared but the right upper zone opacity remained. This raised suspicion for TB and the patient was referred to the TB clinic for further investigation.

This case highlights the fact that you need to look at *everything* on the image, and often go beyond just answering the immediate clinical question.

Figure 12.62 Chest x-ray 8 weeks later

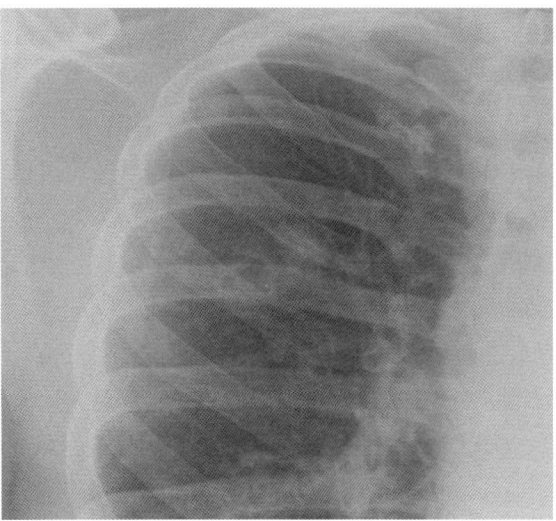

Figure 12.63 Magnification of right upper zone

Case 33

Clinical details: unwell with cough now for several weeks, treated with antibiotics. Query consolidation/pneumonia?

Comment on the image.

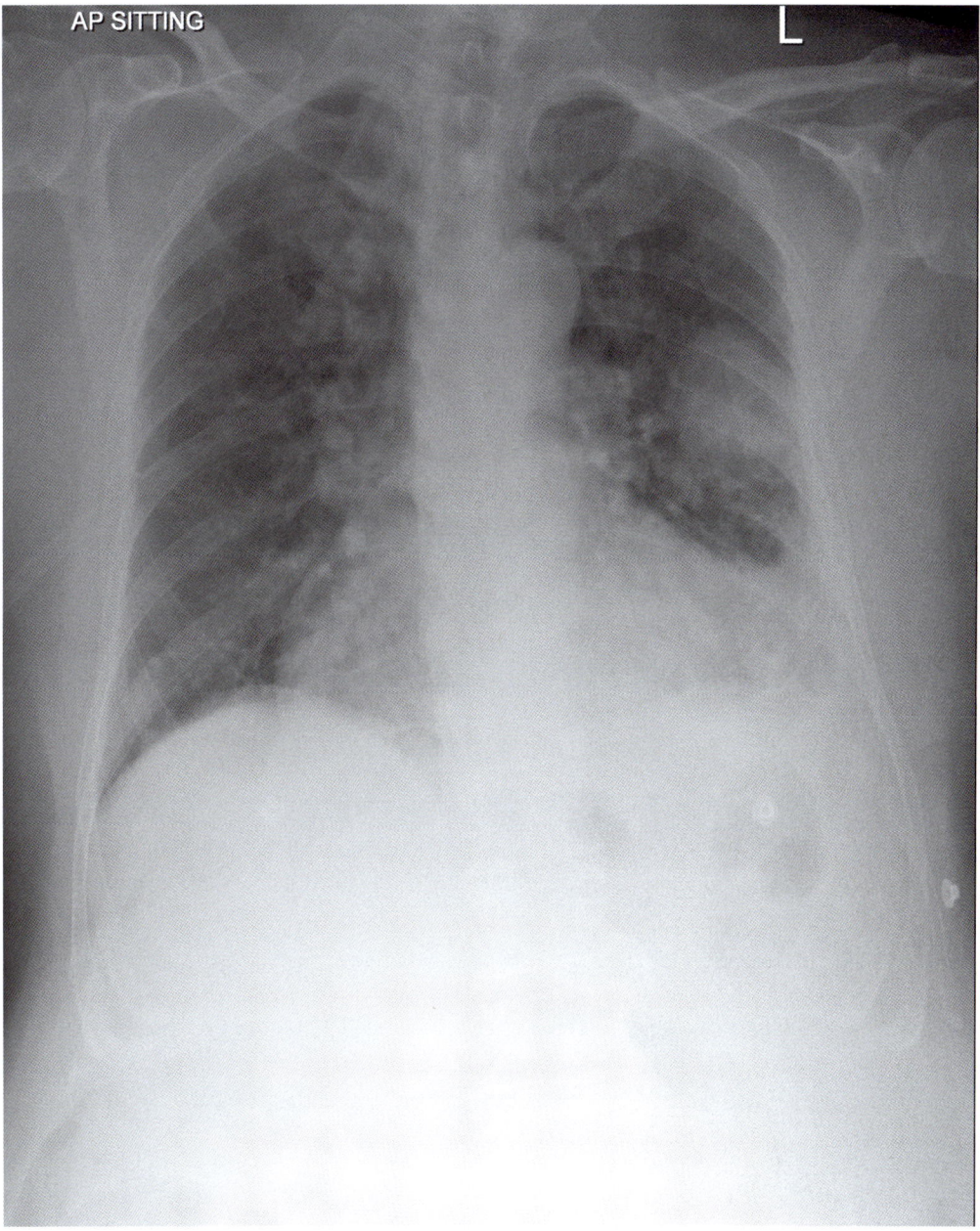

Figure 12.64

Answer to Case 33

There is marked confluent consolidation throughout both lungs, and a large rounded opacity in the left mid zone. Considering the patient's clinical details and the image, it is most likely to be rounded pneumonia. However, a follow-up image 8 weeks after treatment is required to ensure resolution. If the opacity has not improved following treatment, there is concern for a lung cancer.

The heart is enlarged, with a left-sided pericardial fat pad; however, on this image there are no other signs of heart failure. The patient had known ongoing chronic cardiac failure (CCF). Elderly patients may often have evidence of consolidation/pneumonia and CCF on their chest x-ray.

Case 34

Clinical details: heavy smoker with prolonged cough, query lung nodule? Comment on the image.

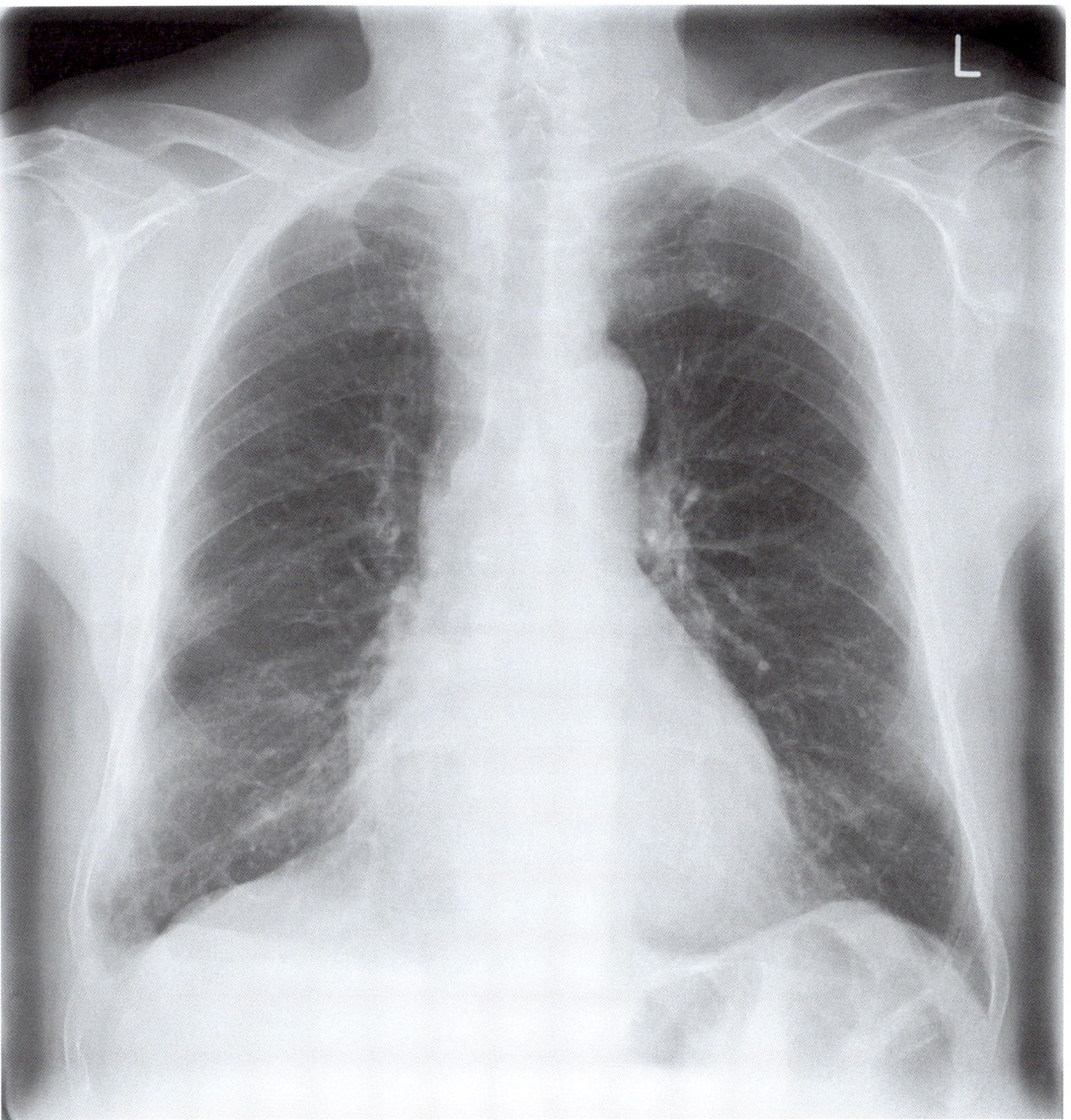

Figure 12.65

Answer to Case 34

There is a left upper zone opacity, which is most likely a lung nodule but it is overlying ribs. The x-ray department the patient was imaged in has a dual energy x-ray machine. Put simply, this machine for one x-ray exposure (very slightly higher dose than normal) has the facility to produce two additional types of images: one demonstrating lung; the other demonstrating bone (almost like subtraction images). This is useful if you are unsure whether the opacity is lung or bony related.

In this case, the dual energy images demonstrated it was a lung nodule. The patient was referred to the lung nodule fast-track service and a HRCT was performed. On other occasions, the dual energy chest x-ray may demonstrate that what appears to be a lung nodule is actually a bone anomaly; hence saving the patient from having a higher-dose CT scan, and answering the clinical question more quickly.

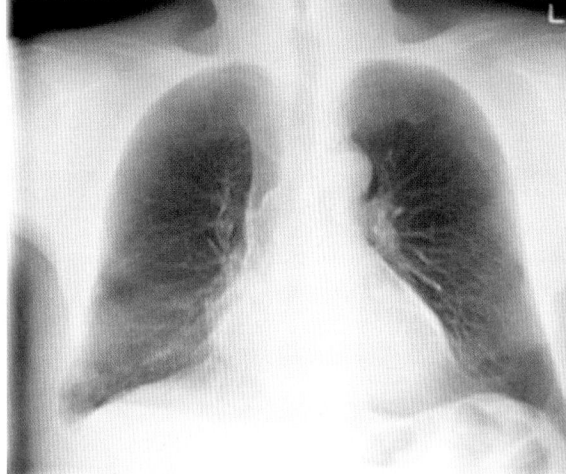

Figure 12.66 Dual energy; lung image

Figure 12.67 Dual energy; bone image

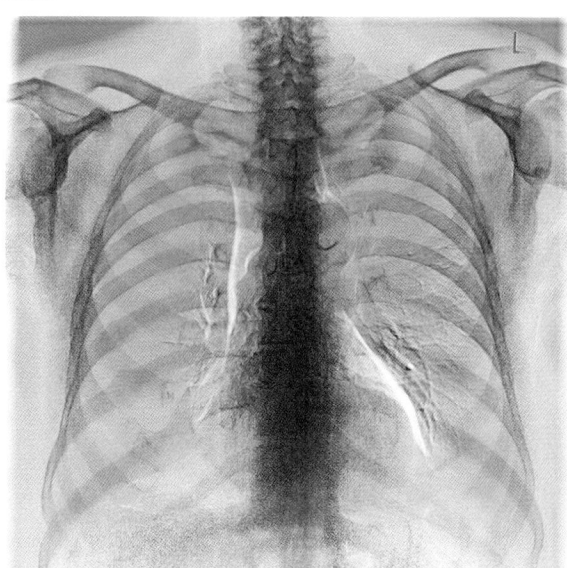

Case 35

Clinical details: heavy smoker, with prolonged cough and haemoptysis. Query lung nodule?

Comment on the image.

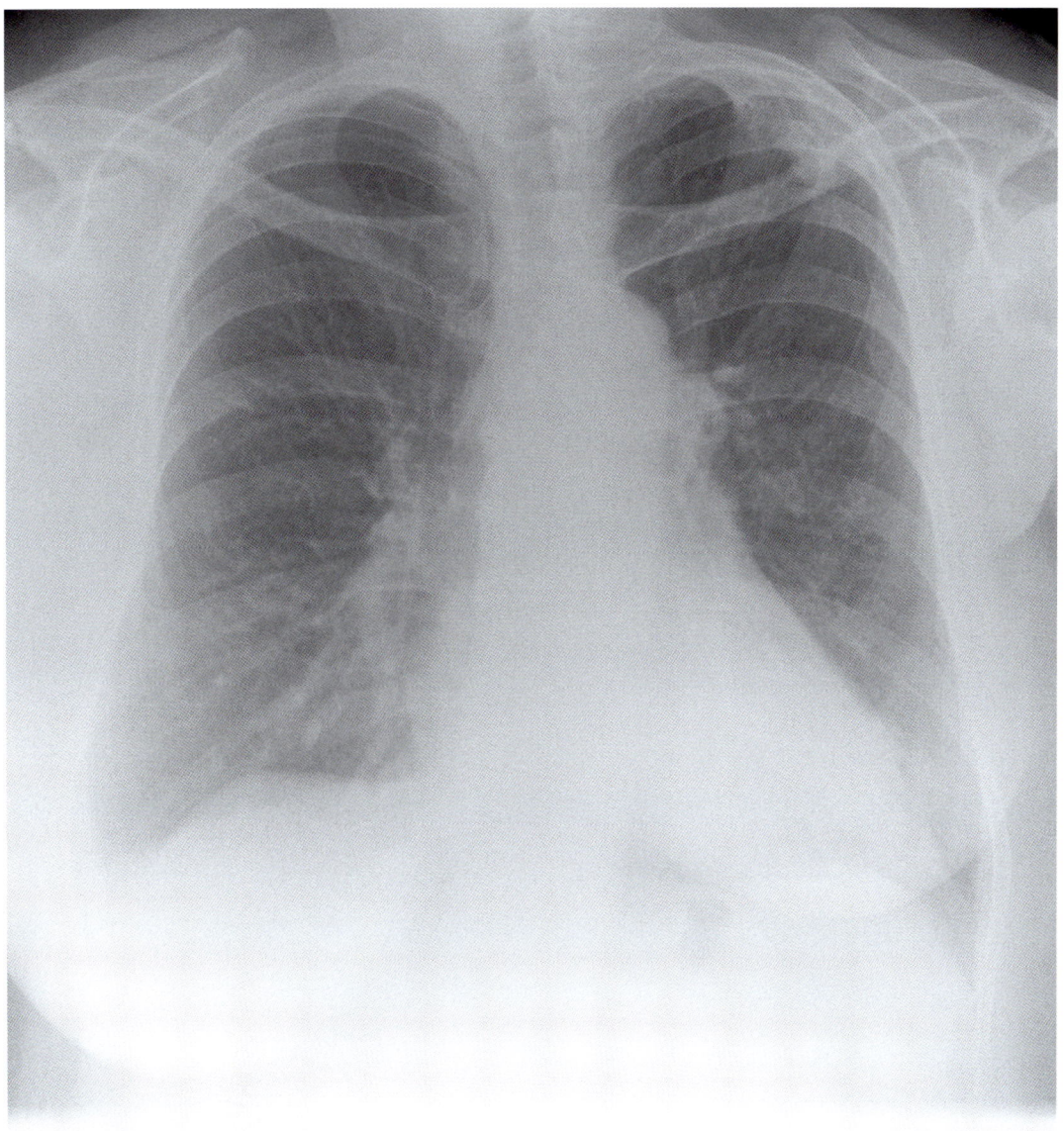

Figure 12.67

Answer to Case 35

Again, there is a left apical opacity, this time overlying the clavicle. The patient was x-rayed in a small remote x-ray department, but additional views can still be done to help further assess the area of concern initially. An apical view was done, which demonstrated the opacity free of the clavicle; it was a lung nodule and the patient went for HRCT.

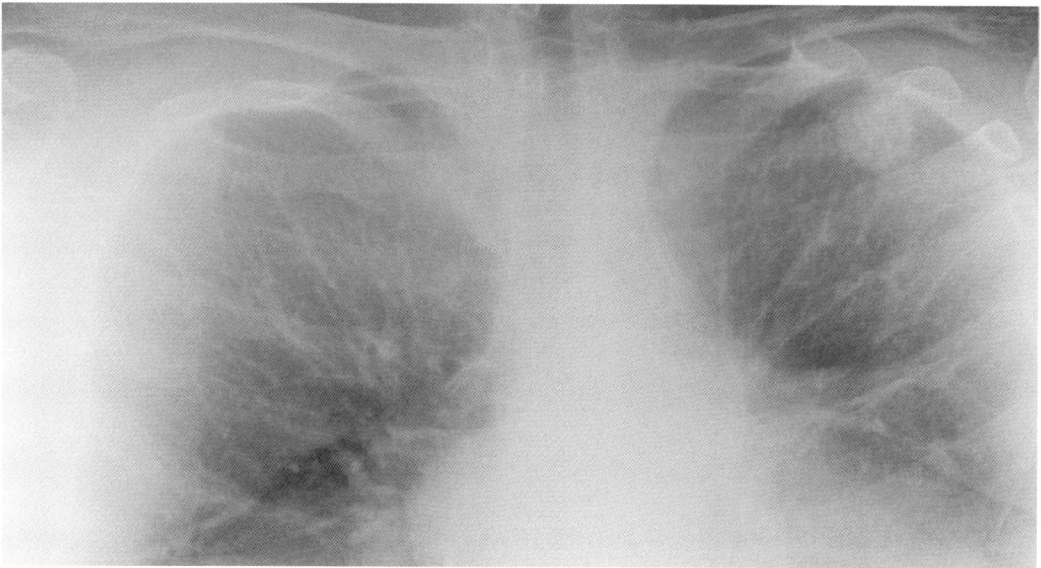

Figure 12.68 Apical view

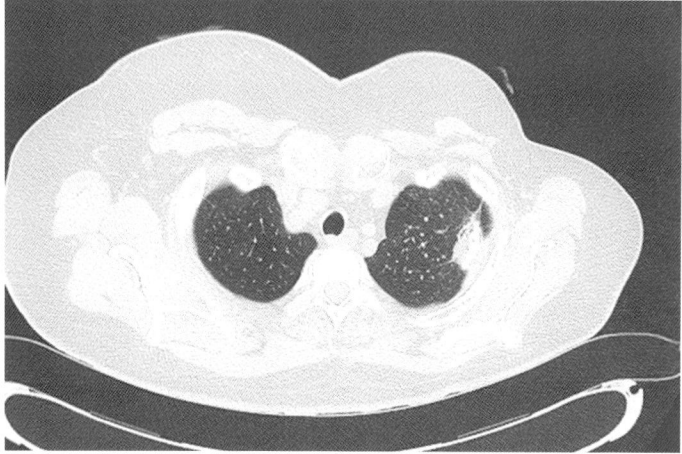

Figure 12.69 HRCT

Case 36

Clinical details: known previous surgery to right acromioclavicular joint. Recent numerous falls, now with chest pain.

Comment on the image.

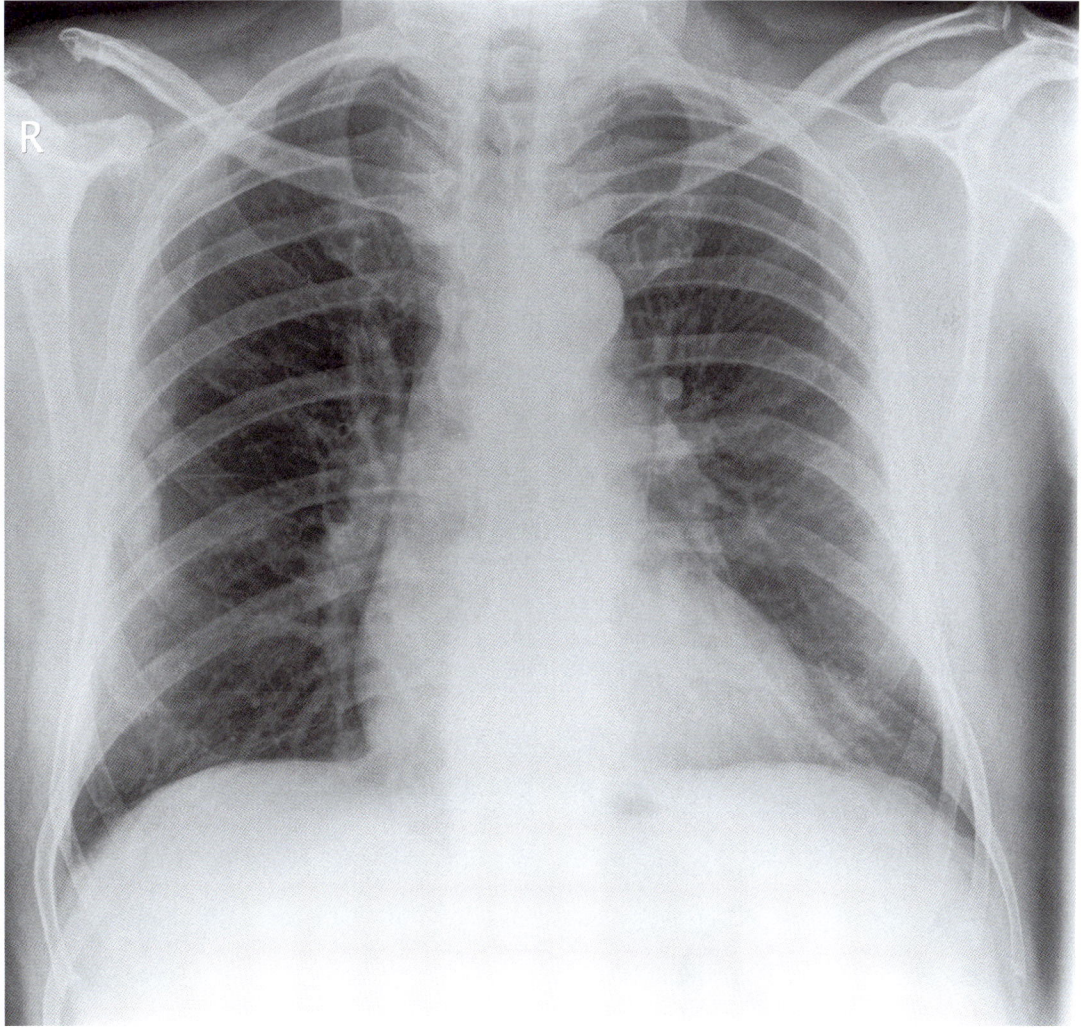

Figure 12.70

Answer to Case 36

There is a right 5th anterior rib anomaly. An oblique view was done of the ribs in this area, and this demonstrated that it was an old healed fractured rib with callous. No acute bony injury was demonstrated on this image. No reason for the patient's falls or chest pains was demonstrated; there were no signs of infection, and no heart failure. Again, this case shows how useful additional projections can be.

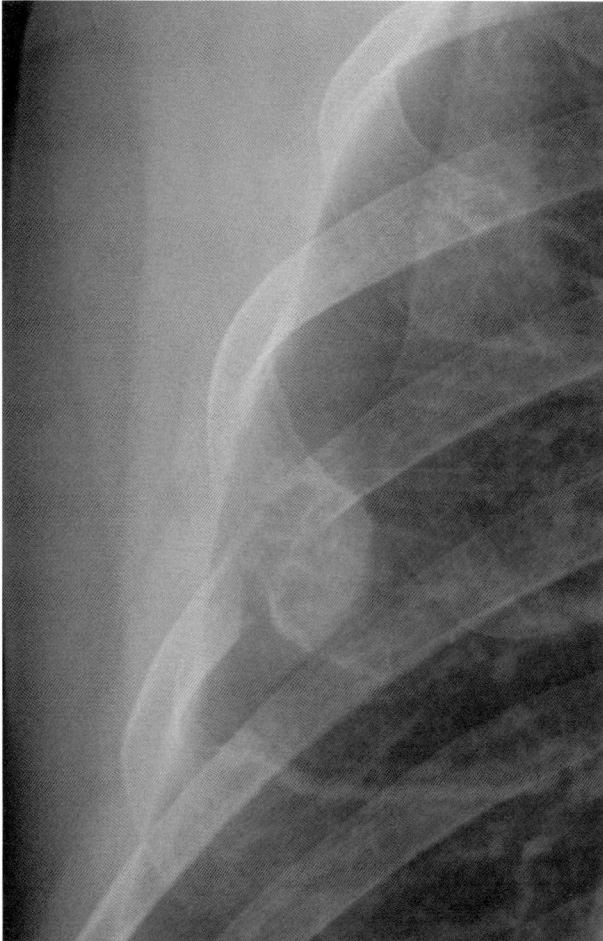

Figure 12.71 Oblique view

Case 37

Clinical details: long-term chest condition, now with increased cough. Query any new consolidation?

Comment on the image.

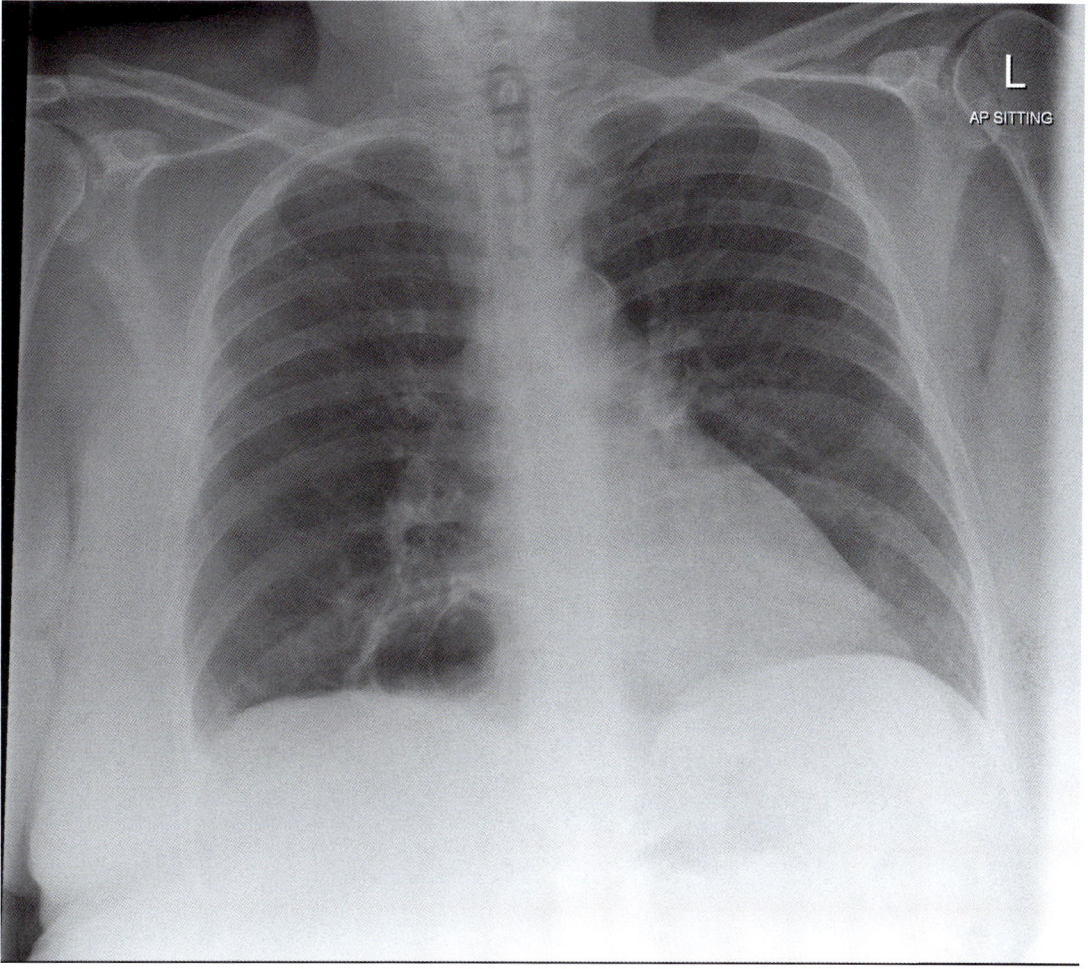

Figure 12.72

Answer to Case 37

At the right cardiophrenic angle there is a cystic area; this is cystic bronchiectasis.

The patient has had bronchiectasis changes for many years. There is no new consolidation present.

Early bronchiectasis changes are often evaluated with HRCT.

Case 38

Clinical details: multiple-injury patient on intensive care. Query adult respiratory distress syndrome? Query pneumothorax?

Comment on the image.

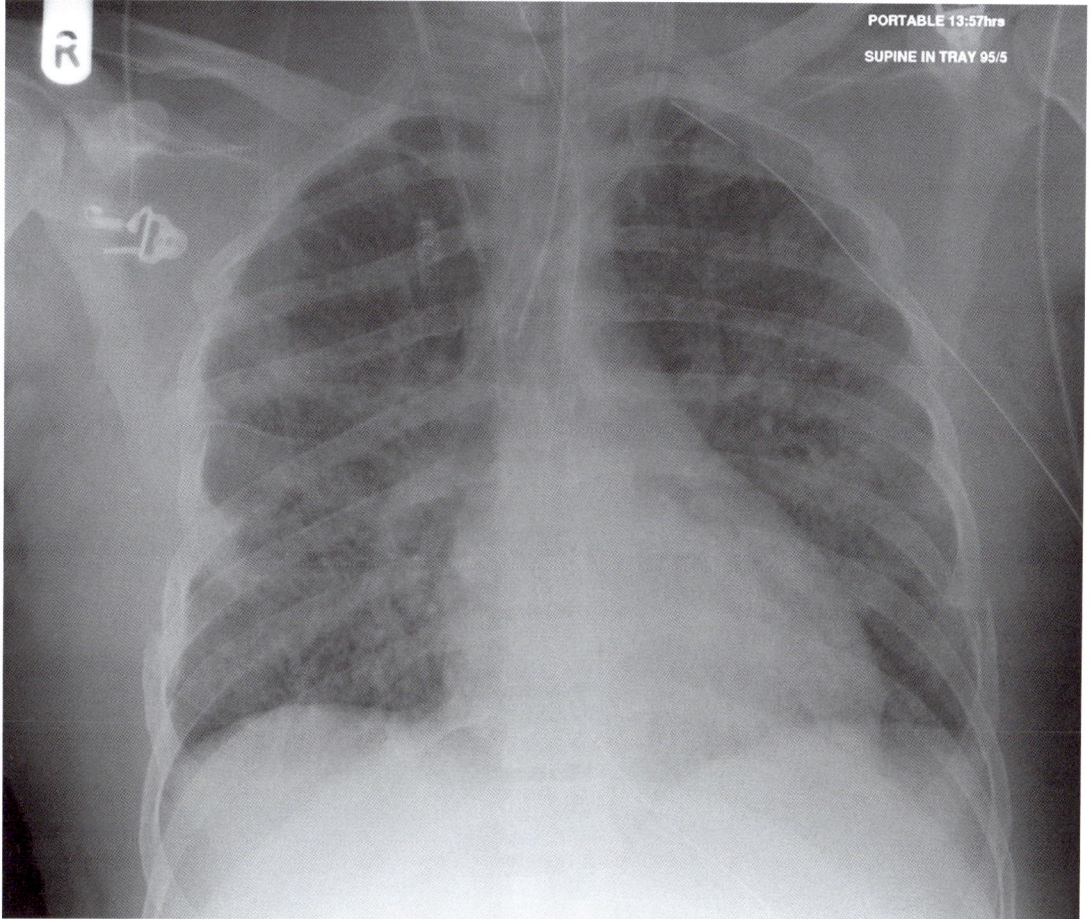

Figure 12.73

Answer to Case 38

There are multiple bilateral rib fractures. There also appears to be bilateral confluent consolidation. In this case it is due to adult respiratory distress syndrome (ARDS) but there can be many different causes and it will often require a diagnosis of exclusion.

The definition of ARDS is:
- Radiographic infiltrates
- Reduced PaO_2/FiO_2
- Normal left atrial filling pressure.

Most of the defining characteristics of ARDS are therefore clinical findings, rather than radiographic ones. However, it is useful to see an example of an ARDS x-ray to store in our brain's image library of chest conditions!

This image does not demonstrate a pneumothorax, but they are sometimes difficult to see on the supine patient. See Cases 22 and 23 for examples of pneumothorax in the supine patient.

Case 39

Clinical details: returned from a long time in Asia, cough, night sweats, generally feeling unwell.

Comment on the image.

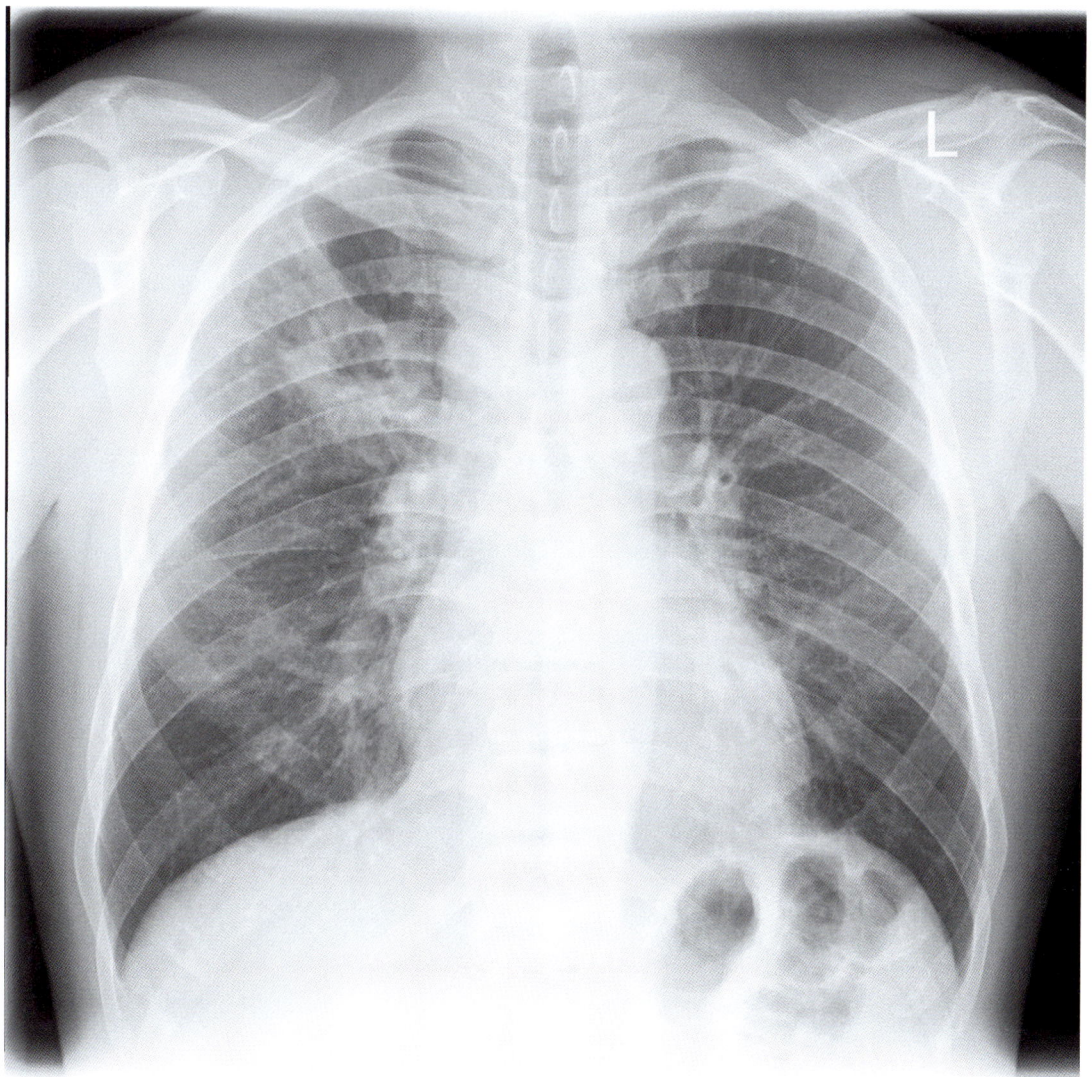

Figure 12.74

Answer to Case 39

There is right upper zone consolidation, with what appears to be a cystic area or abscess in the middle of it. It is common to have consolidation with cavitation in TB, which is what is occurring on this image. There is also widening of the right upper mediastinum and hilar lymphadenopathy. In primary TB, lymph node enlargement occurs in about 95% of cases (the rate is lower in post-primary TB).

Appearances are consistent with TB and fit with the clinical details.

Please compare with Case 32, which was suspected TB.

Case 40

Clinical details: patient fell onto left side, now painful with difficulty breathing. Comment on the image.

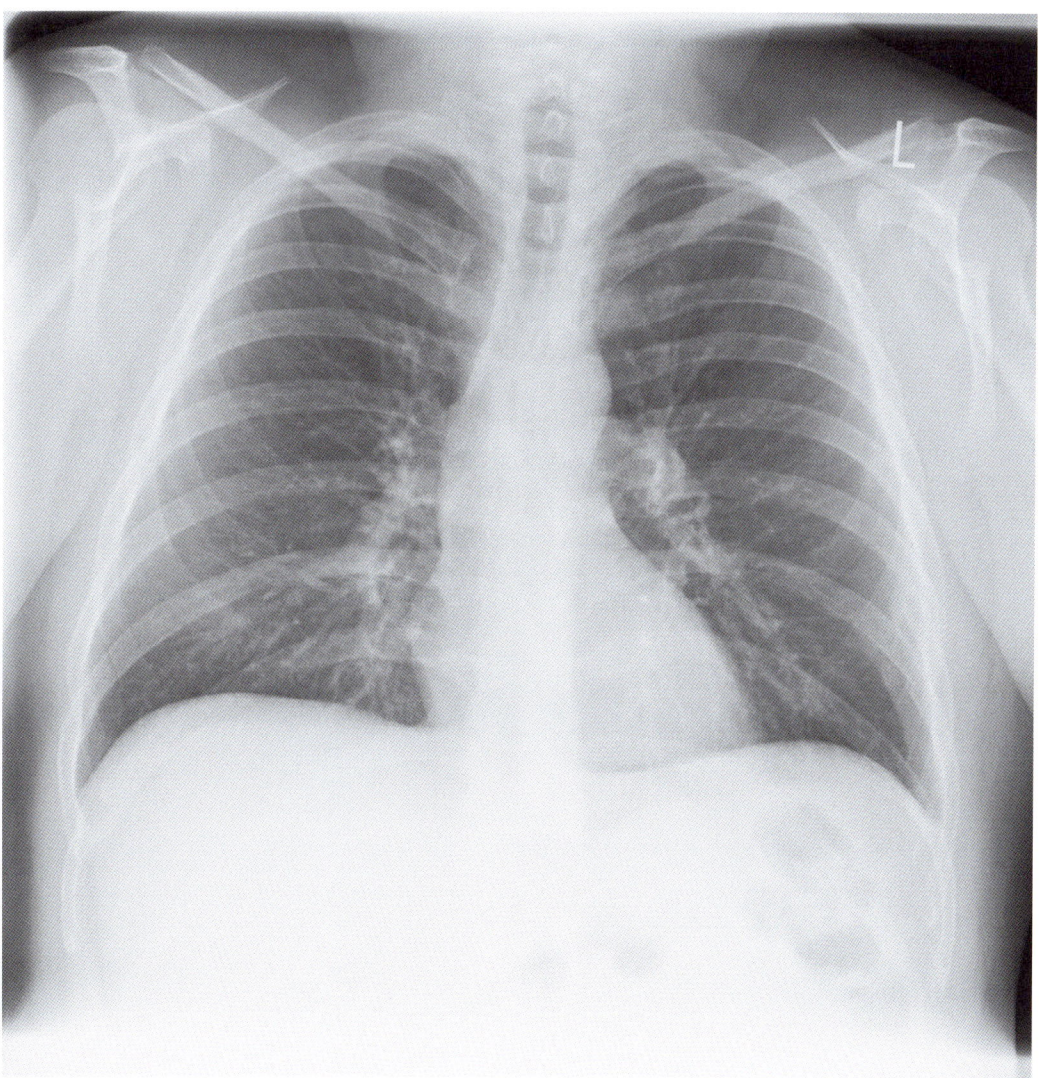

Figure 12.75

Answer to Case 40

There are fractures of the left 8th and 9th posterior ribs with a small haemothorax. No other bony injury demonstrated.

Another chest x-ray was taken several weeks later, and the patient now appears to have a large pleural effusion. This is most likely to be due to an increased haemothorax, as a result of the previous injury.

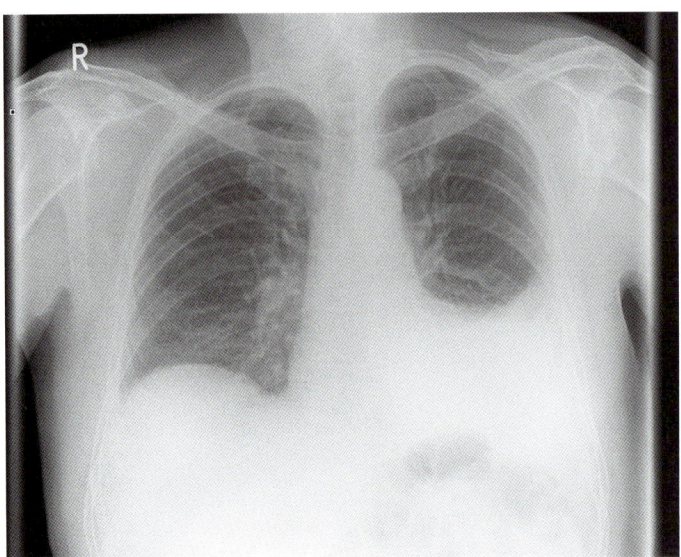

Figure 12.76

It always amazes me that what looks like a small pleural effusion or haemothorax is actually a large amount of fluid within the lung, which is why the patient struggles to breathe. I think this is better demonstrated in a diagrammatic form; so the above patient probably started with 200–300ml of fluid in their left lung and now has close to 2 litres in their left lung.

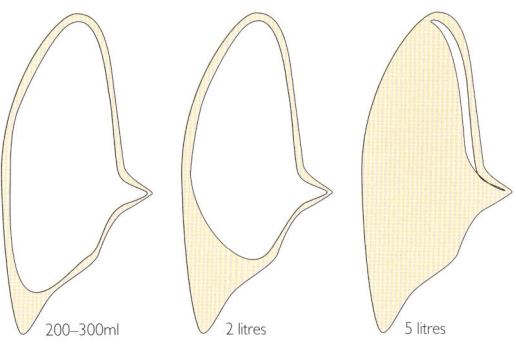

Figure 12.77 Pleural effusions

Case 41

Clinical details: hoarse voice, cough and breathless, haemoptysis.

Comment on the image.

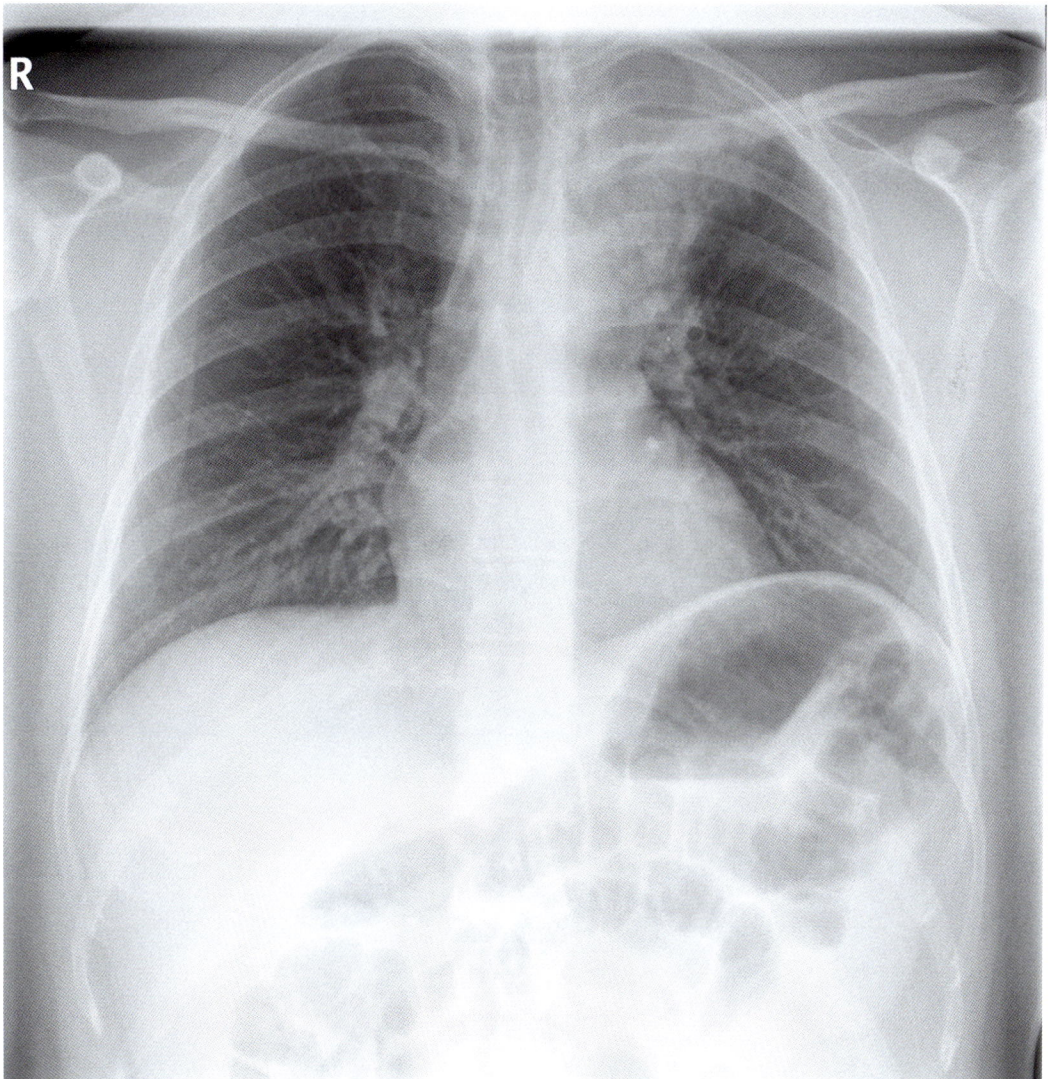

Figure 12.78

Answer to Case 41

There is a left apical mass, which has resulted in loss of definition of the left upper heart border (think silhouette sign) due to increased density of the mass and associated consolidation. There is also loss of the lung markings at the left apex.

This was a Pancoast's tumour, which fits with the radiographic appearances and the clinical details.

Case 42

Clinical details: patient has previously had severe multiple injuries. Today crackles at right base, query right-sided chest infection?

Comment on the image.

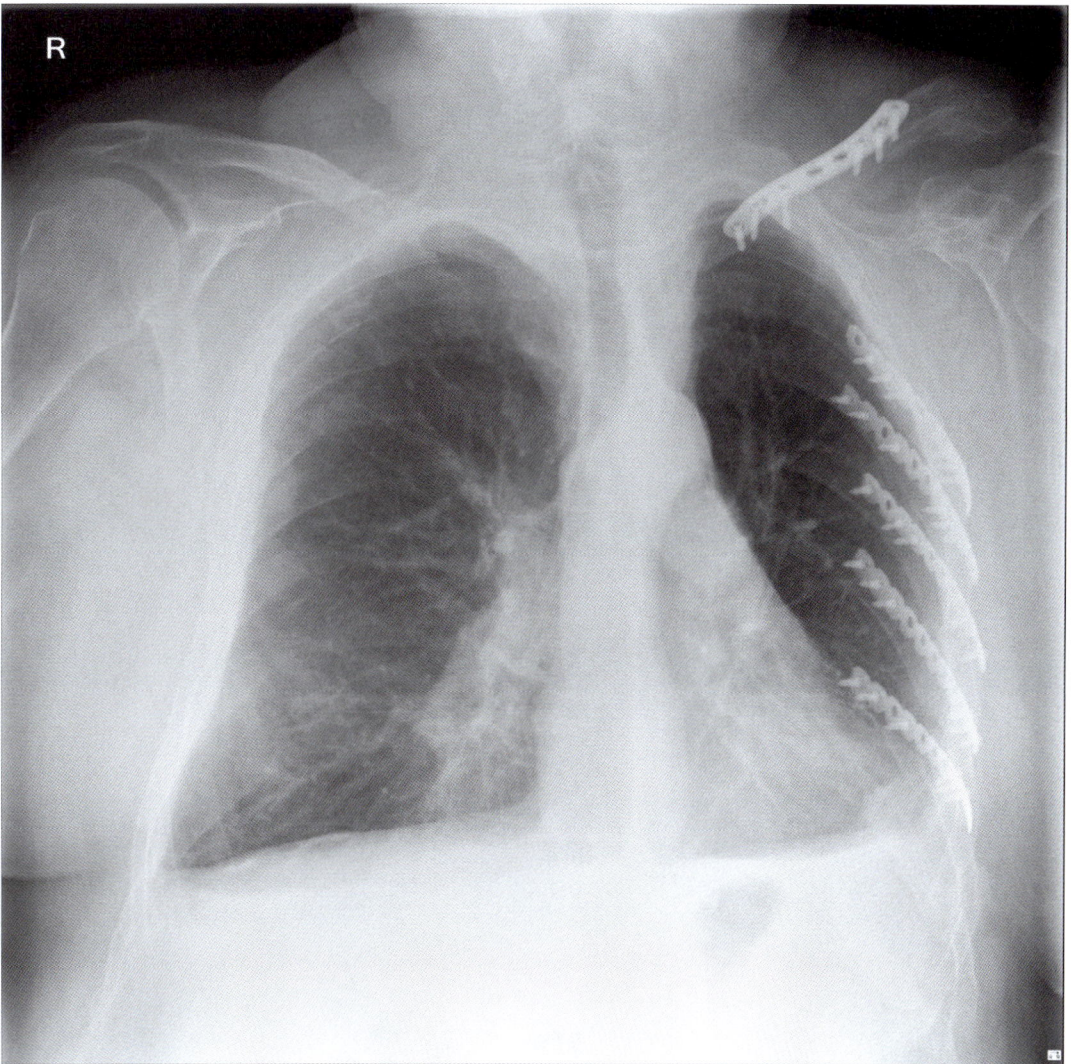

Figure 12.79

Answer to Case 42

What is initially noted is previous fractures to the left clavicle and left ribs, with open reduction and internal fixation (ORIF) of five left ribs and the clavicle. This appears to have resulted in some loss of left lung volume and pleural thickening at the left costophrenic angle, probably at the site of an old haemothorax. The right lung appears clear, with no consolidation or collapse demonstrated. Image was consistent with previous.

It is noted that both diaphragms are flattened, with coarse broncho-vascular markings and overinflated right lung (which may be due to COPD). There are also some subtle pleural plaques along the right hemidiaphragm, which are consistent with previous asbestos exposure.

Case 43

Clinical details: patient x-rayed in resuscitation room after road traffic collision, with severe difficulty in breathing.

Comment on the image.

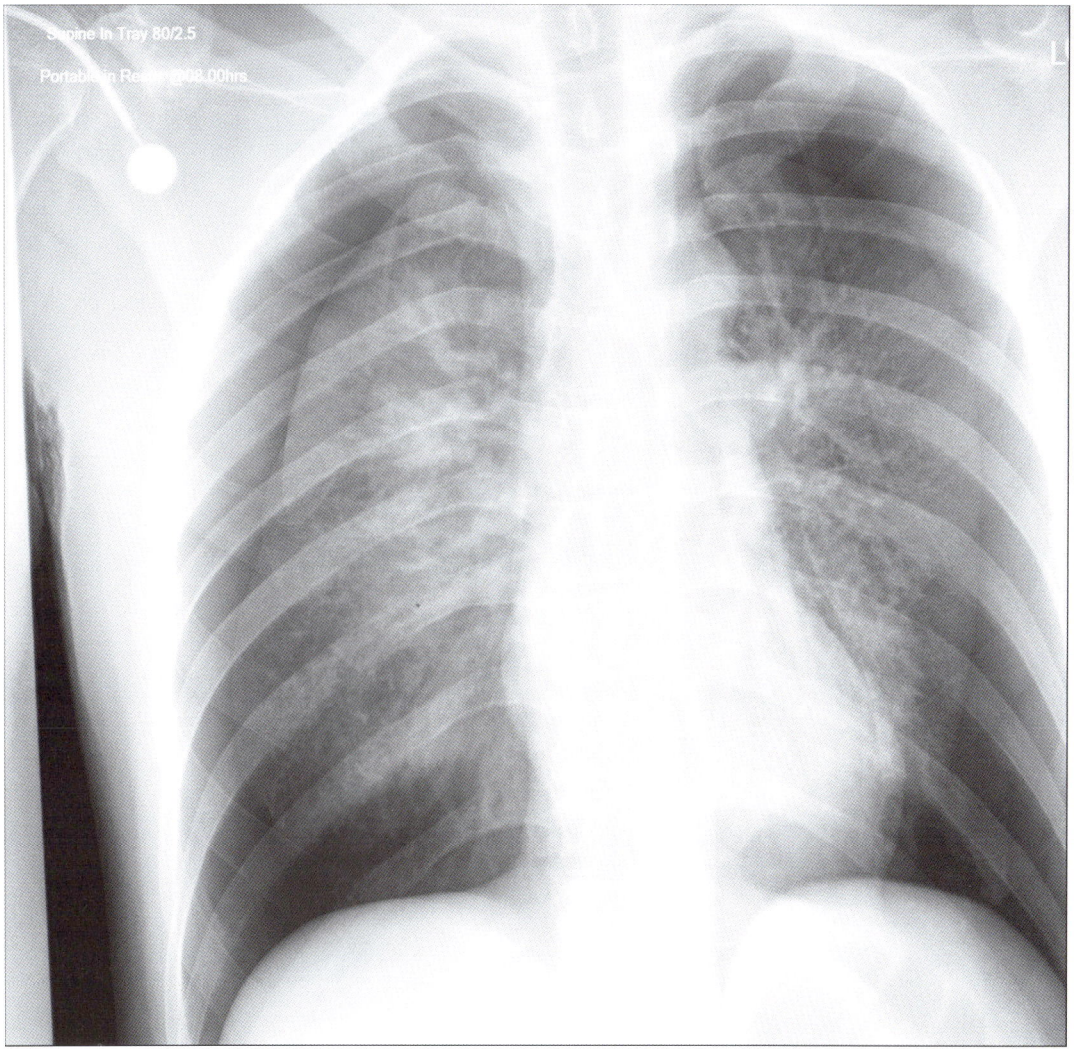

Figure 12.80

Answer to Case 43

There are unusually large bilateral pneumothoraces, with no lung markings demonstrated lateral to the collapsed lungs.

Case 44

Clinical details: known drug user, has fever and cough. Query chest infection? Comment on the image.

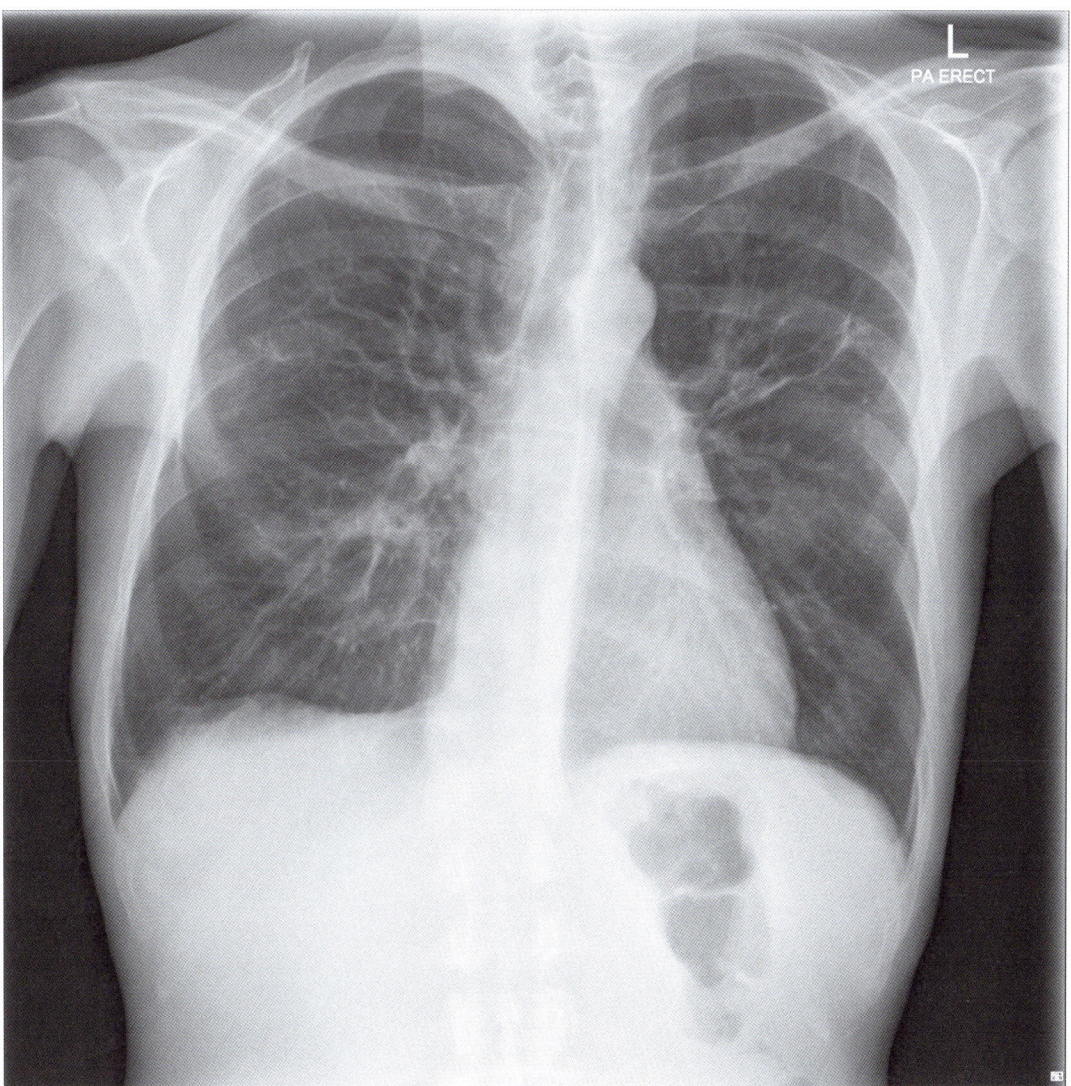

Figure 12.81

Answer to Case 44

There is no new consolidation or collapse. However, there are increased lung markings and chronic lung changes, including bullae in both upper zones, which were present on previous images.

Case 45

Clinical details: increased difficulty breathing, query cause?

Comment on the images.

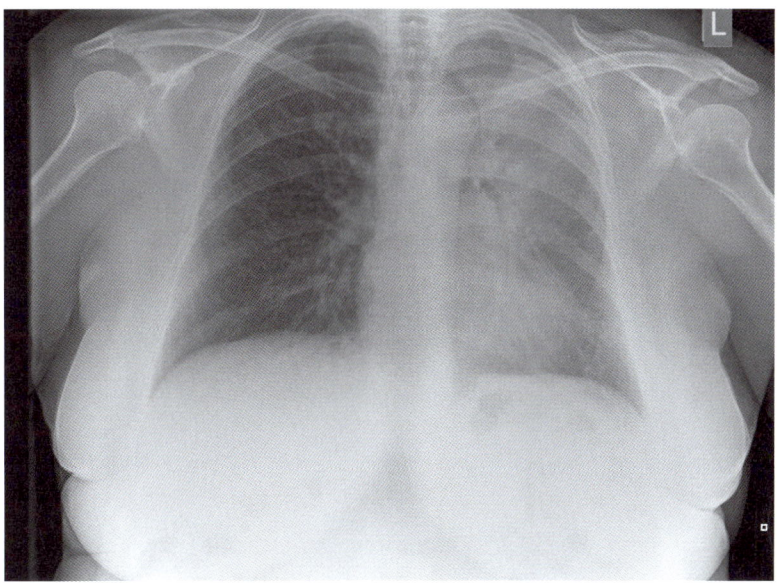

Figure 12.82

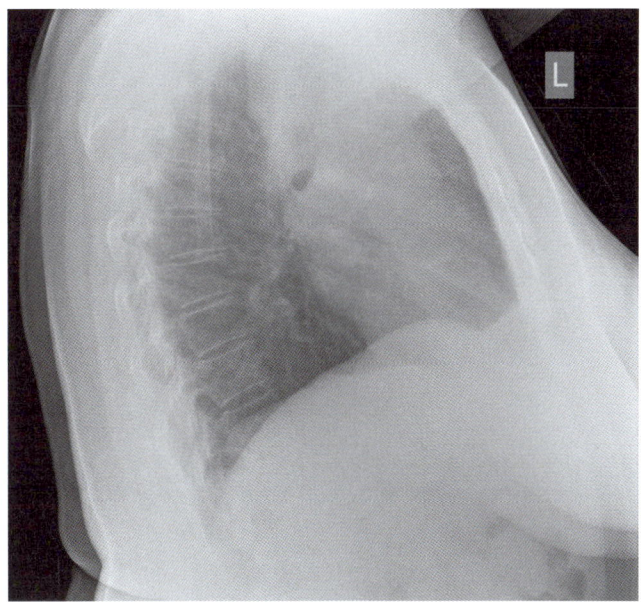

Figure 12.83

Answer to Case 45

Compare with Case 18.

There is left upper lobe collapse, demonstrated by loss of the clear definition of the left upper mediastinum/heart shadow, and a veil-like appearance of the left lung. In this case we also have a lateral view, which demonstrates very clearly the left upper lobe collapse.

This appearance may be caused by a mucous plug, or a mass blocking off the airway. Further investigation with HRCT is required.

Case 46

Clinical details: heavy smoker, loss of weight, cough, haemoptysis. Comment on the images.

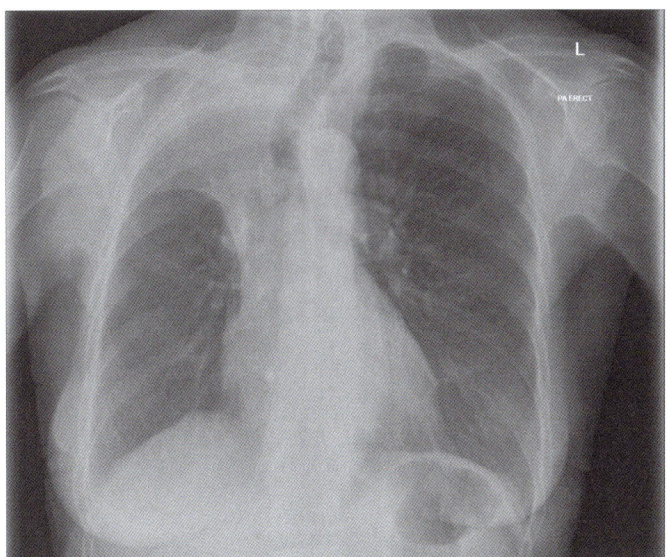

Figure 12.84

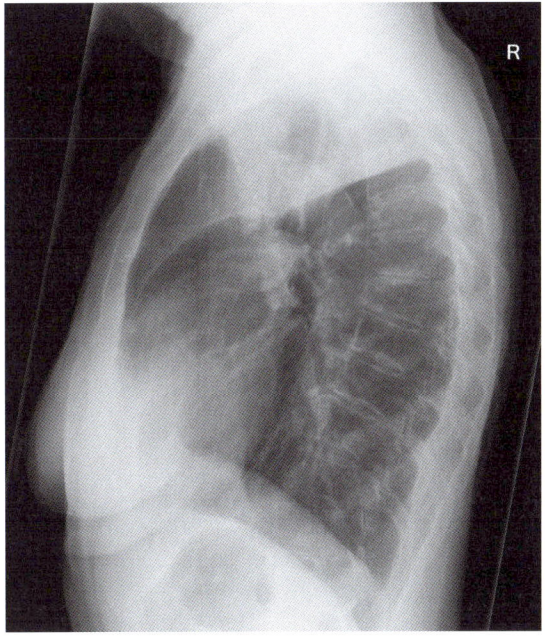

Figure 12.85

Answer to Case 46

Compare with Case 28.

Already, reading the clinical details, one is highly suspicious of lung cancer. The images demonstrate right upper lobe collapse, with the mediastinum and trachea moving towards the right to take up the space left by the collapsed lung. A large mass is also demonstrated at the right hilar. The lateral view clearly demonstrates the right upper lobe collapse. Compare the lateral view of this case with the lateral of the previous one. Both demonstrate upper lobe collapse but of different lungs; see how they differ.

Case 47

Clinical details: long-time heavy smoker, cough, with some difficulty in breathing. Query COPD?

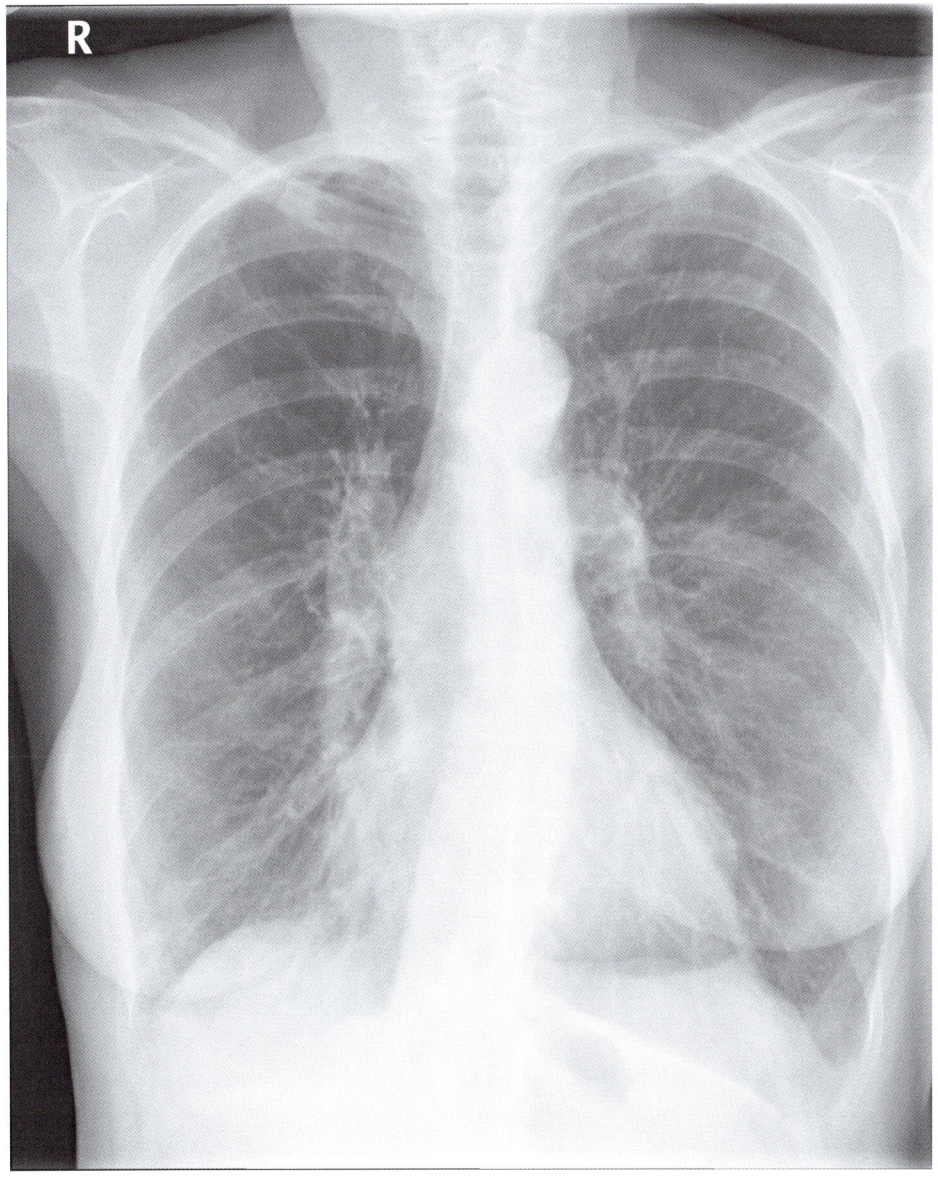

Figure 12.86

Answer to Case 47

The lungs are overinflated, with flattened diaphragms and slight tenting of the left diaphragm. There are coarse broncho-vascular markings. The appearances are consistent with COPD. Bilateral nipple shadows also demonstrated.

Case 48

Clinical details: young female just returned from 6 months in India. Extremely unwell with severe difficulty breathing.

Comment on the image.

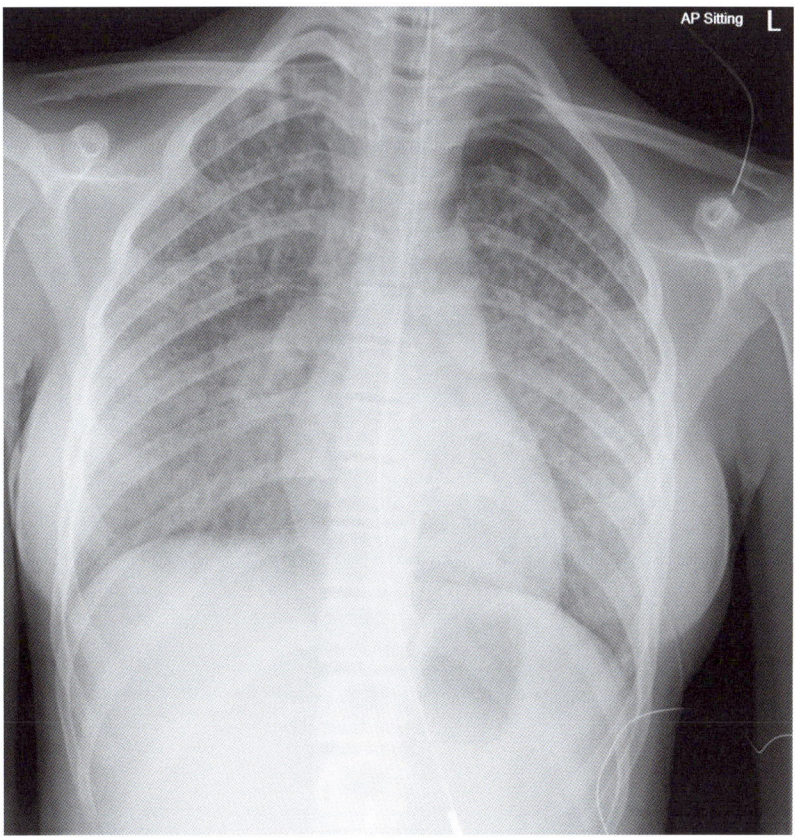

Figure 12.87

Answer to Case 48

There is a left-sided apical pneumothorax.

There is generalised intrapulmonary shadowing, made up of a myriad of tiny dots in all areas of the lungs. These dots resemble millet seeds, which is why this condition is known as miliary tuberculosis. These miliary densities will normally be 0.5–20mm in diameter, sharply defined and usually involve the apices first. Miliary TB results from haematogenous dissemination of the disease.

Case 49

Clinical details: cough and fever. Query chest infection?

Comment on the image.

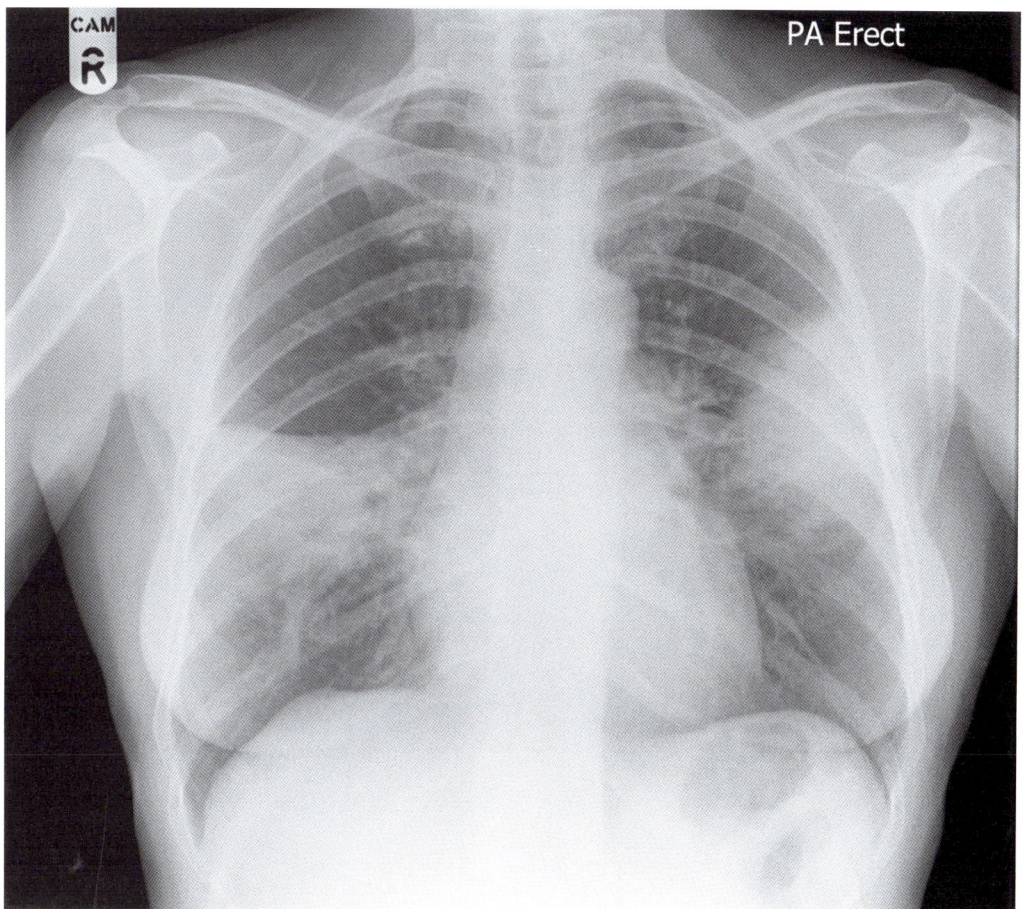

Figure 12.88

Answer to Case 49

There is bilateral mid zone wedge consolidation, most likely from an infective process. Suggest treat as infection, with repeat x-ray after 6–8 weeks to ensure resolution of appearances.

Case 50

Clinical details: Cough and fever. Query chest infection?

Comment on the image.

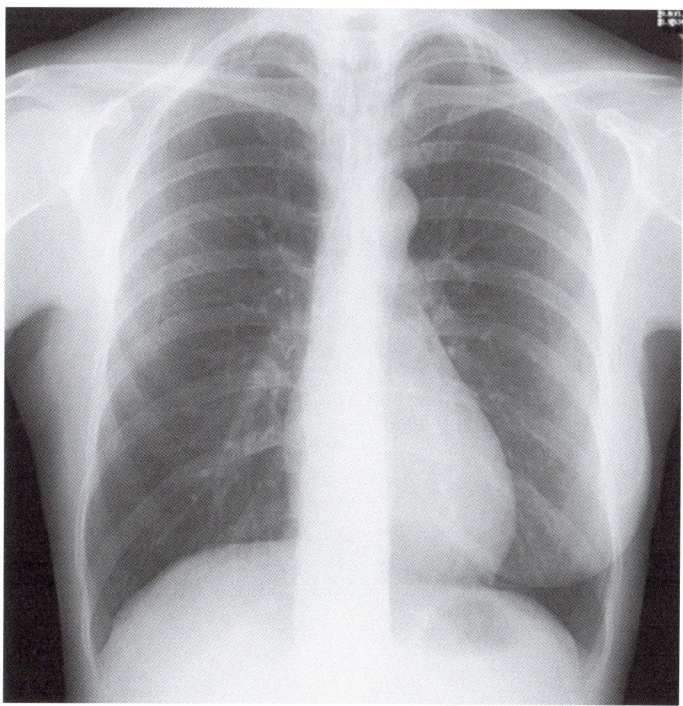

Figure 12.89

Answer to Case 50

There is no consolidation or collapse, and no sign of a chest infection. The lungs and pleura are clear. The heart and mediastinum are normal.

This is in fact a normal chest x-ray, which is sometimes the most difficult report to do in chest imaging, for fear of missing something.

Case 51

Patient has had a productive cough, with some left-sided chest pain. Query respiratory tract infection?

Has previous medical history of plasmacytoma.

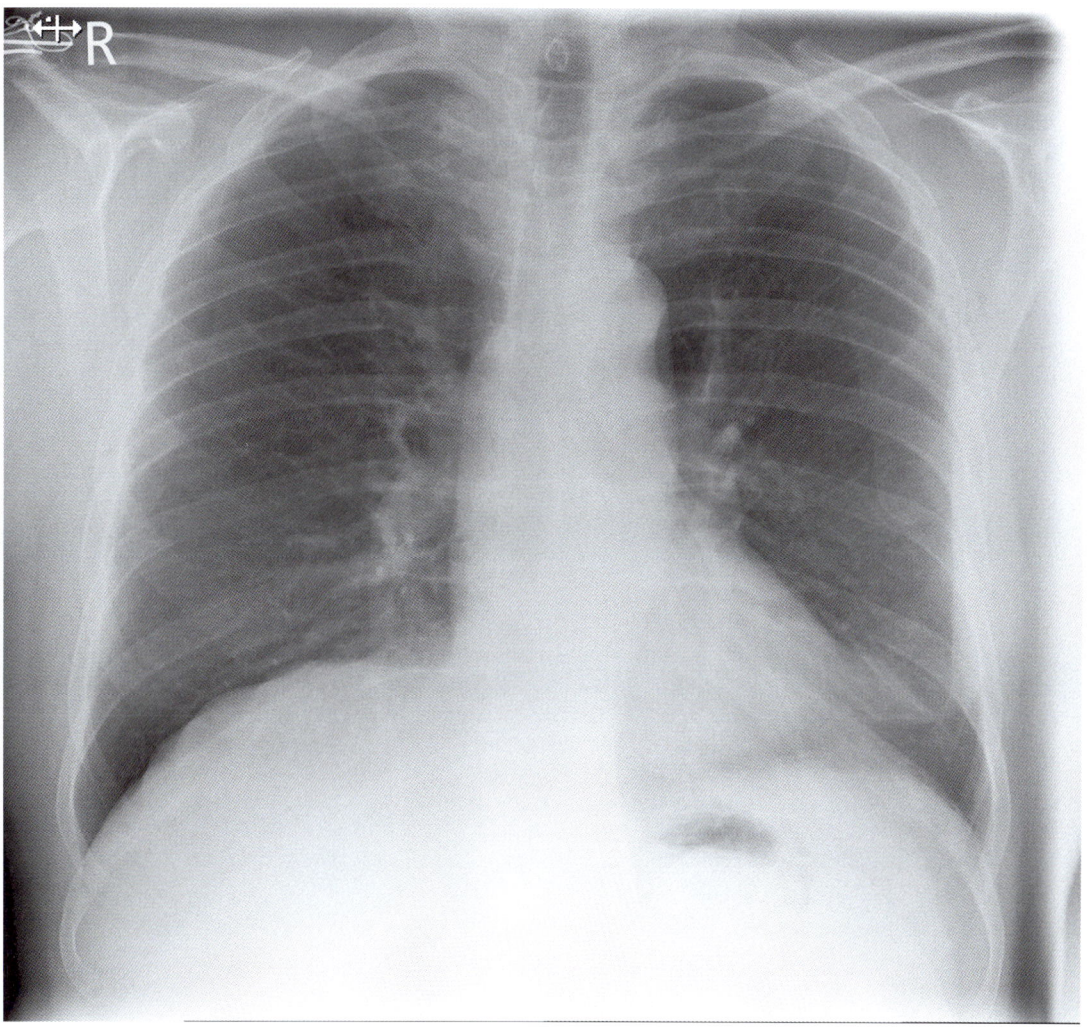

Figure 12.90

Answer to Case 51

There is loss of the clear definition of some of the left heart border with increased opacification of the left lower zone. Considering the clinical details, this is most likely to be due to consolidation from an infective process. A follow-up x-ray after 6–8 weeks should be advised, following appropriate treatment, to ensure resolution of appearances.

However, what is perhaps more interesting is the medial aspect of the right clavicle. It is not clearly defined on this image (the cortex is not clear) but there is a lytic area medial clavicle. Dedicated shoulder images were requested; and on further investigation it was found to be a plasmacytoma.

This highlights the importance of reviewing everything on an image. On a chest x-ray, remember to review the bones, and on musculoskeletal images remember to review the soft tissues, and chest if included. Also, remember the clinical details should help you, and you should answer the clinical question posed; but don't let the clinical details stop you from looking at everything on the image. As in this case, you might be concentrating so hard on answering the clinical question regarding an infection that you don't look for bony lesions. On the original request, it did not mention plasmacytoma; this was added to assist you. You should therefore always have a system, so there is less chance of missing a pathology.

The shoulder views demonstrate the plasmacytoma more readily at the medial aspect of the clavicle, as well as previous acromion fracture repair.

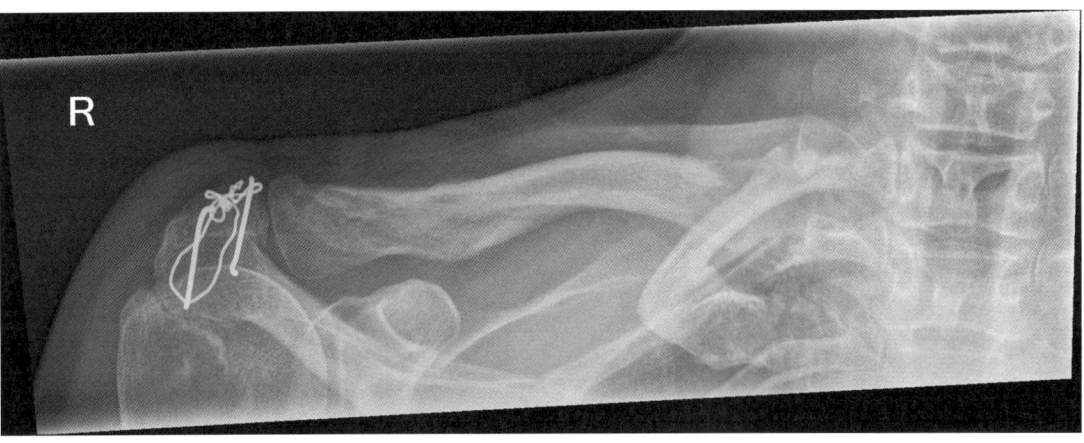

Figure 12.91

Case 52

Patient has been in an RTC.

Comment on the shoulder image. What should be done next?

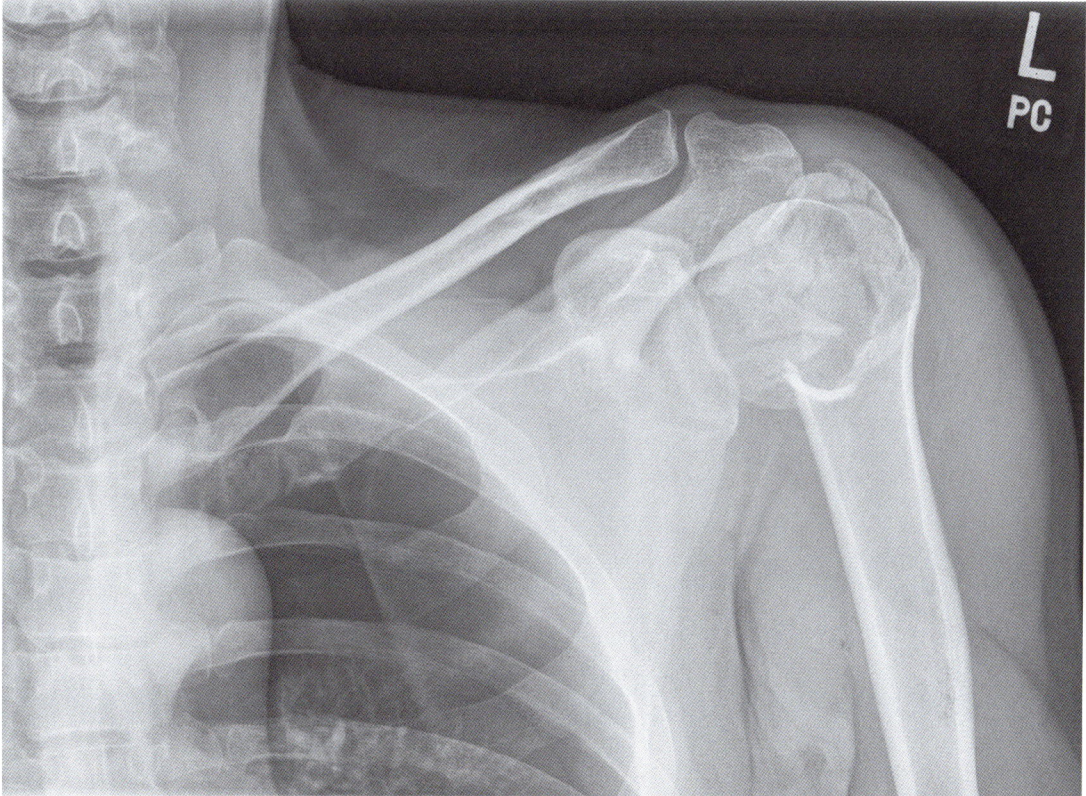

Figure 12.92

Answer to Case 52

There is a severely comminuted fracture of the humeral head, with probable posterior dislocation of the humeral head (although it requires a modified axial to confirm the latter). There is a large pneumothorax, which requires a chest drain.

In answer to the question, if the patient is already in the x-ray department, a chest x-ray should be done, to see the extent of the pneumothorax, and to check for other chest injuries. Depending on the departmental protocols and clinical review, a trauma CT may be done to assess for other injuries, and check the extent of the chest injuries. Also, another view of the shoulder is required (modified axial) to confirm the posterior dislocation.

Case 53

Clinical details: Increased breathlessness and chest pain. Query chronic cardiac failure?

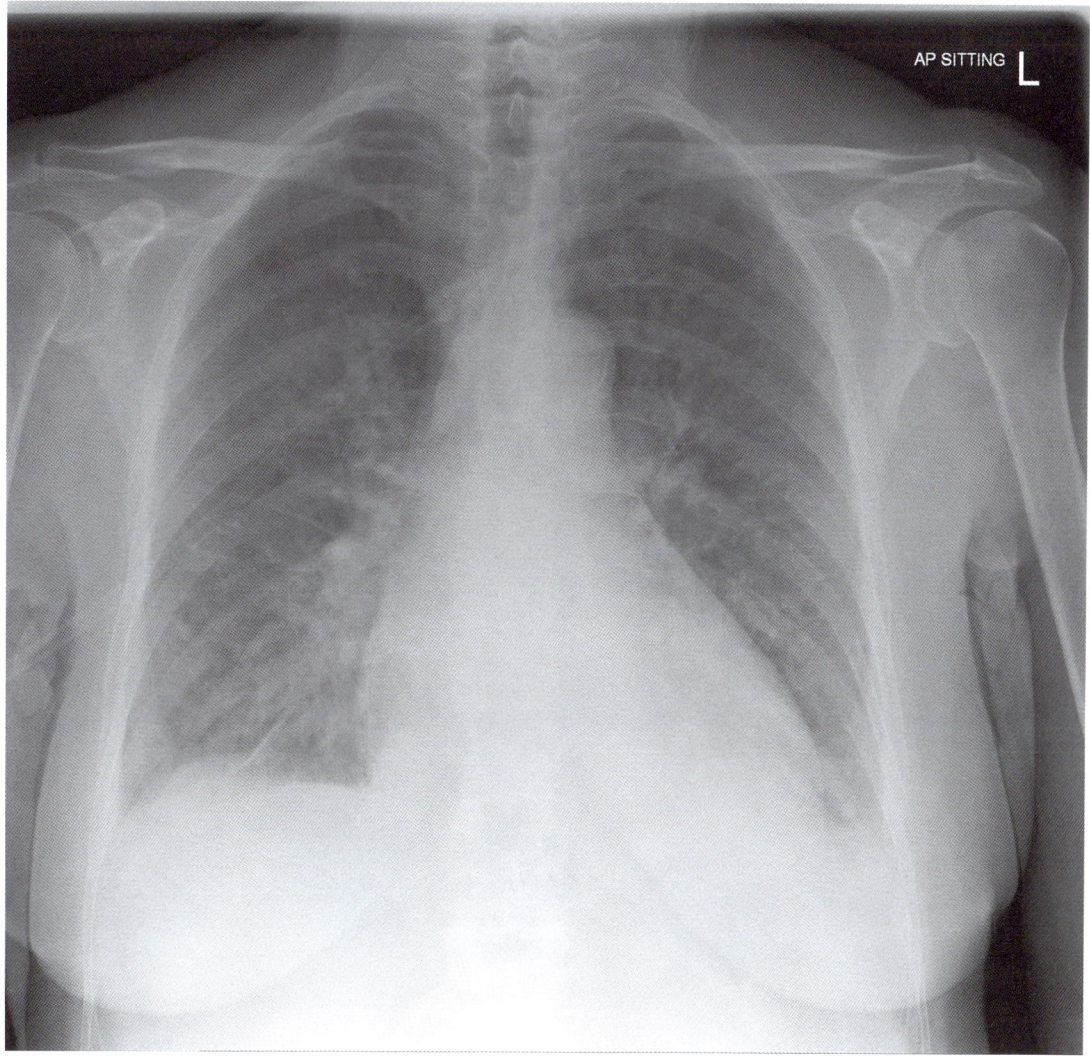

Figure 12.93

Answer to Case 53

There is cardiomegaly, and at this stage it is useful to measure the cardiothoracic ratio and state it. There is interstitial oedema in both lungs – most marked around the hilar region. There is also a left-sided pleural effusion; and probably a small right basal effusion. Appearances are consistent with chronic cardiac failure.

Case 54

Clinical details: follow-up chest x-ray of previous patient. Ongoing chest pain. Query resolution of cardiac failure following treatment?

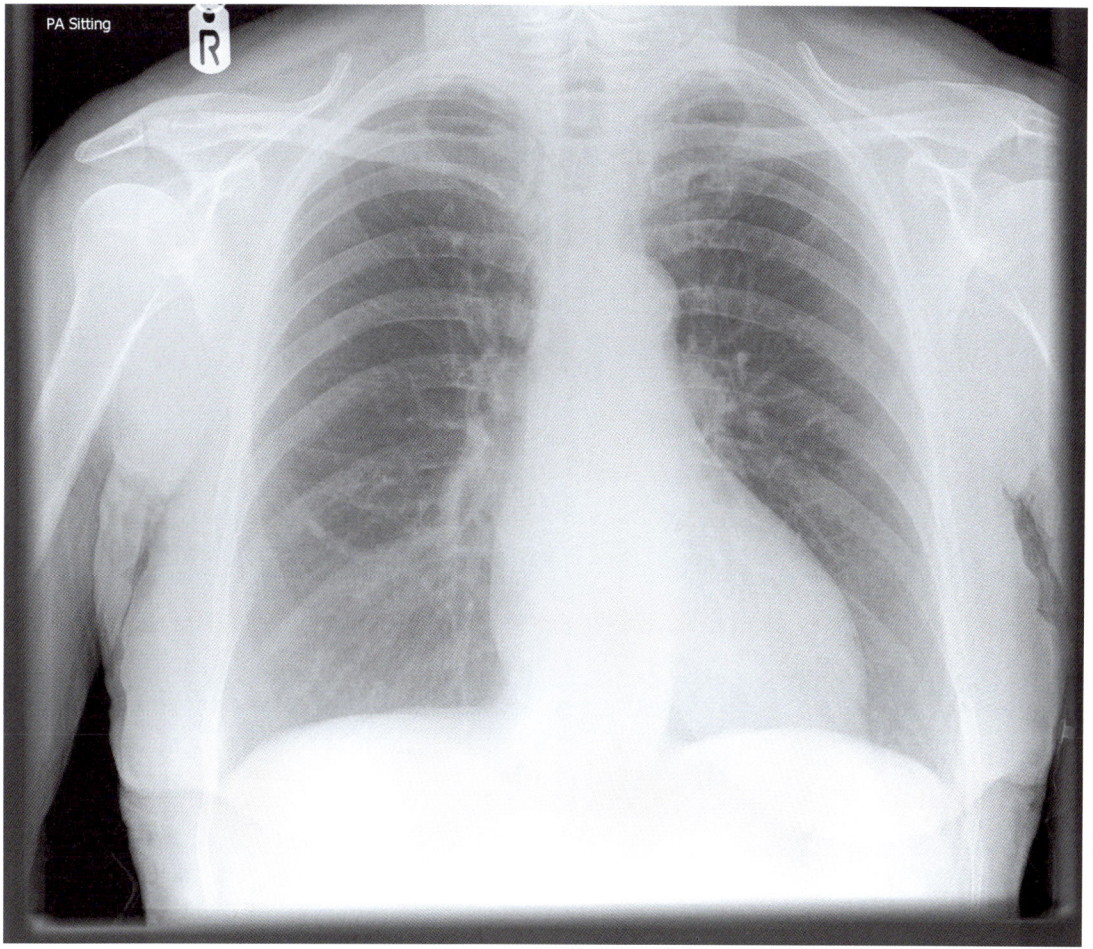

Figure 12.94

Answer to Case 54

There is no cardiac failure, as the x-ray shows normal heart size, no pleural effusion, no interstitial oedema, and no upper lobe vessel diversion. Even now it always amazes me how quickly, with treatment, cardiac failure can sometimes clear from a chest x-ray.

However, there is a right 9th posterior rib fracture which may be the cause of the ongoing chest pain. This was also visible on the previous image/case.

Case 55

Clinical details: known ongoing heart failure, patient had a series of falls recently. Chest pain.

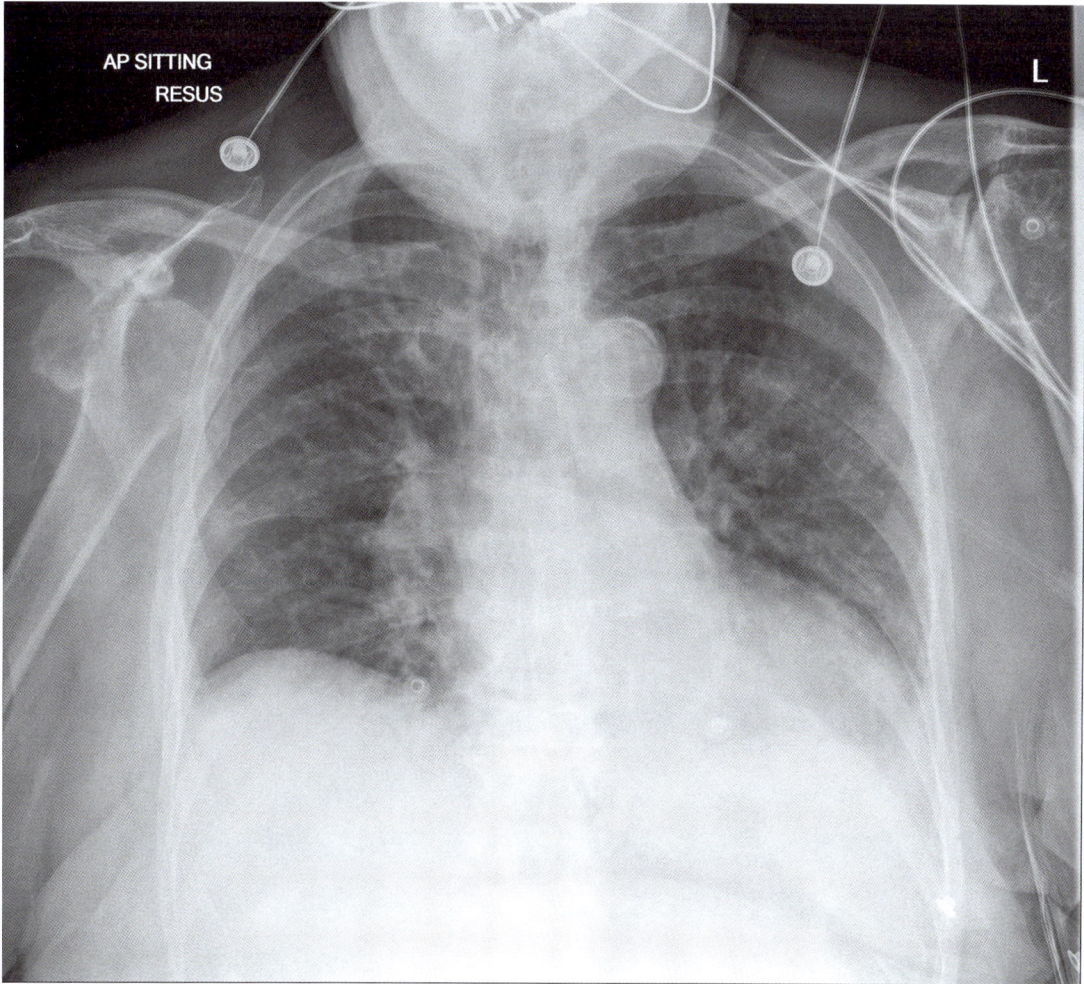

Figure 12.95

Answer to Case 55

There is cardiomegaly, probably a left-sided pleural effusion and interstitial oedema, which is consistent with ongoing cardiac failure. There is also some bronchial wall thickening and the patient had known bronchiectasis.

There is a right anterior humeral head dislocation with 4th to 7th right posterior rib fractures. These are a result of the patient's recent falls and they require treatment.

Case 56

Clinical details: resuscitation patient, chest pain.

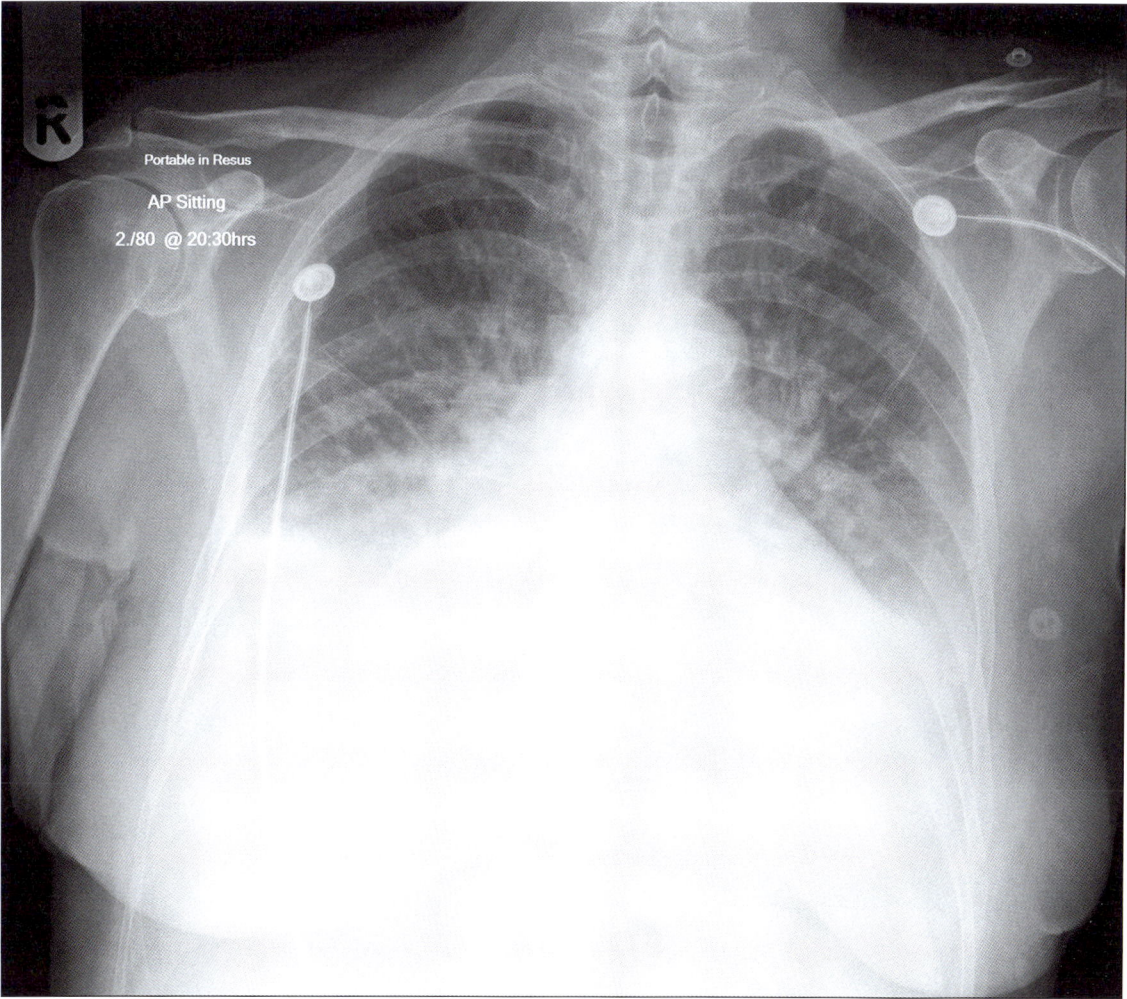

Figure 12.96

Answer to Case 56

The clinical details are fairly basic; but, realistically, this is often all we are given, especially when the patient is in the resuscitation room.

There is cardiomegaly, bilateral basal pleural effusions and marked interstitial oedema in both lungs; all these appearances are consistent with cardiac failure.

Case 57

Young male patient with generalised aching of body and feeling unwell.

Comment on the image.

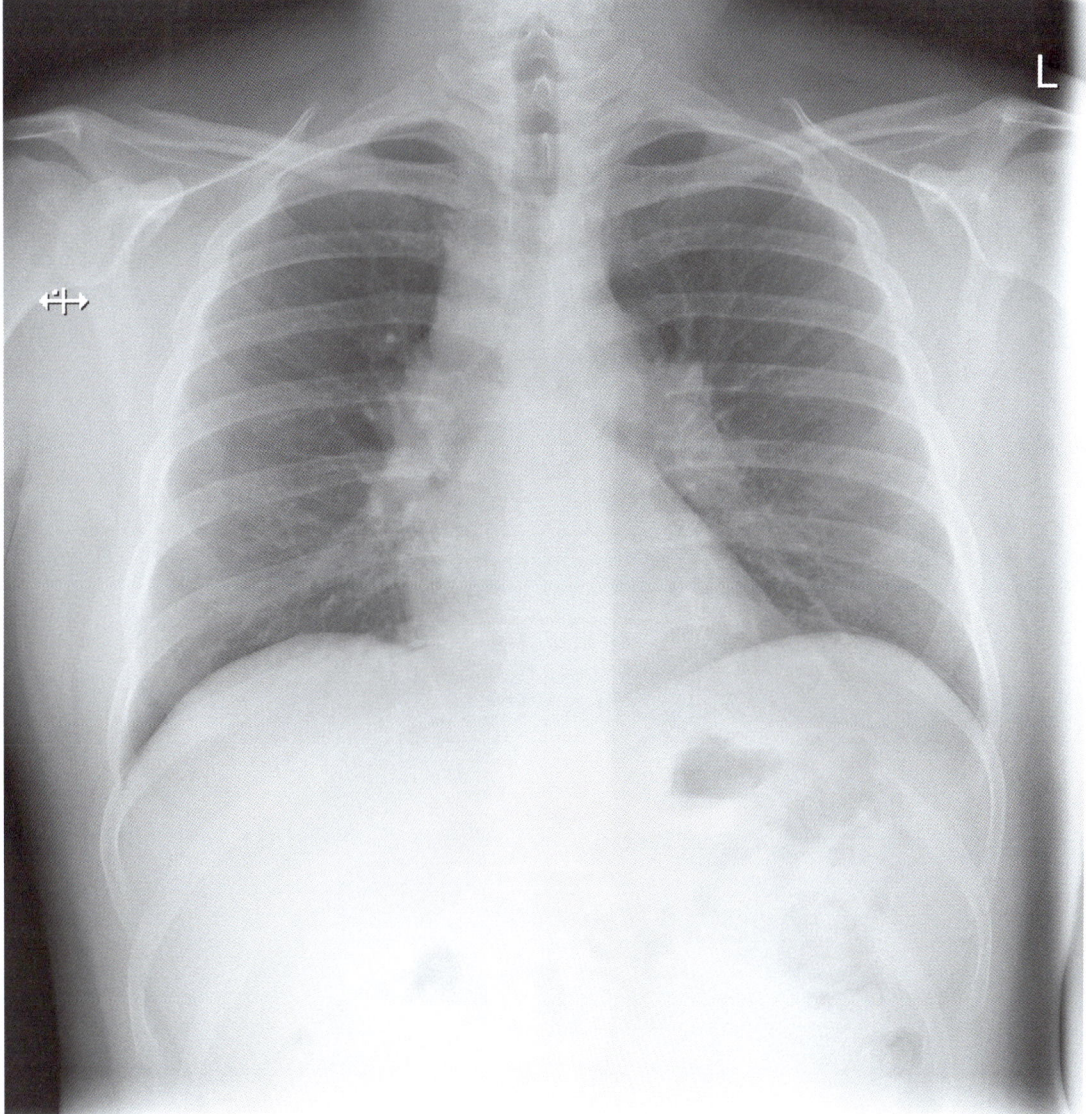

Figure 12.97

Answer to Case 57

There is marked widening of the mediastinum and hilar lymphadenopathy. The lungs are clear. The differential diagnosis in a young patient is lymphoma and sarcoid. The patient often has an HRCT to investigate further. In this case it was found to be sarcoid.

Case 58

Clinical details: heavy smoker with known COPD. Ongoing cough, worse with chest pain.

Comment on the image.

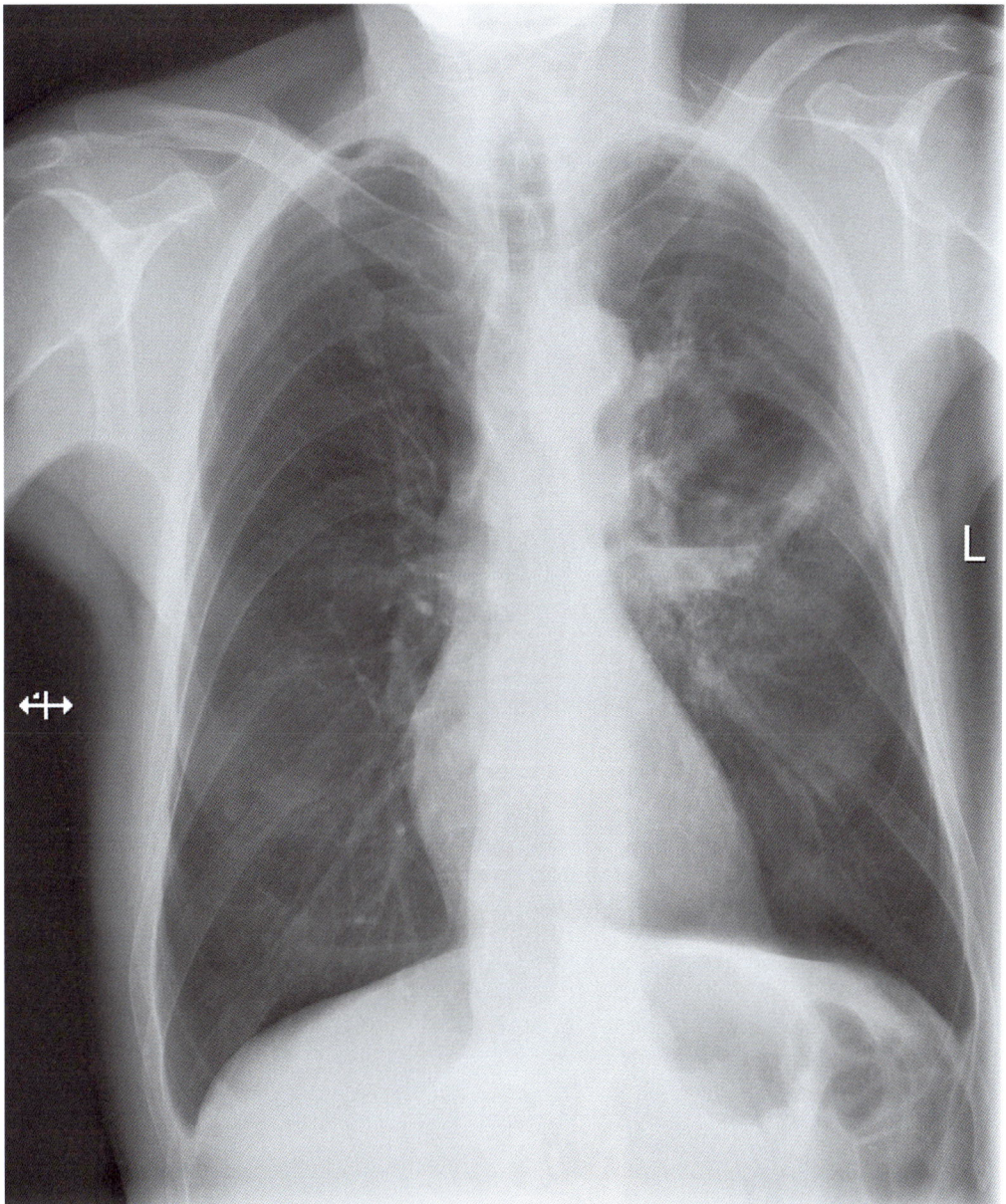

Figure 12.98

Answer to Case 58

The lungs are overinflated with coarse broncho-vascular markings consistent with known COPD. However, there is a large cavitating lesion in the left mid zone. This is most likely to be a cavitating malignancy and requires HRCT and referral to the lung MDT.

Case 59

Clinical details: patient in RTC, chest pain.

Comment on the image.

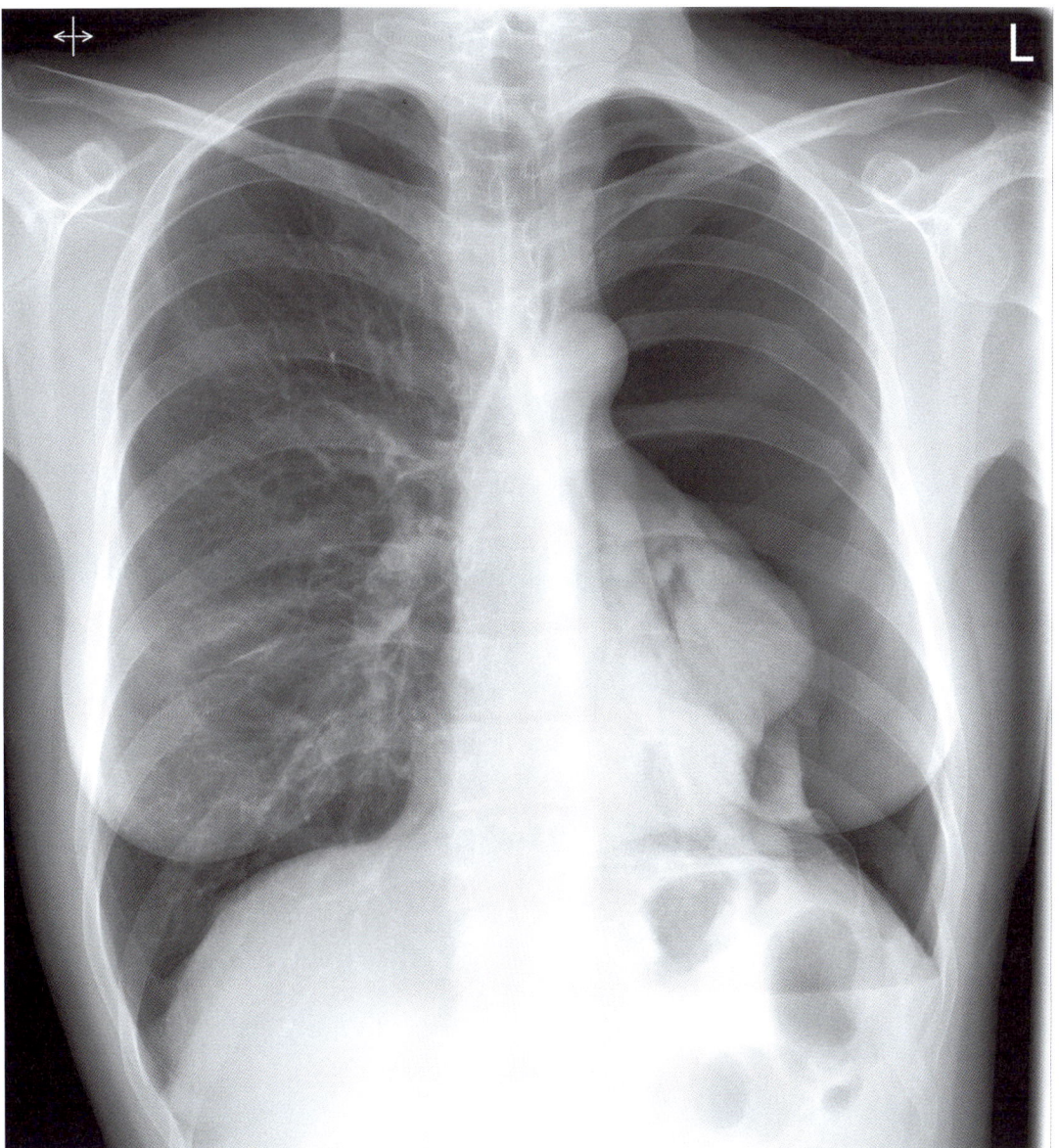

Figure 12.99

Answer to Case 59

There is a complete left-sided pneumothorax. Also noted are left posterior 6th and 7th rib fractures. The patient needs a chest drain.

Case 60

Clinical details: routine follow up chest x-ray for previous consolidation. Comment on the image.

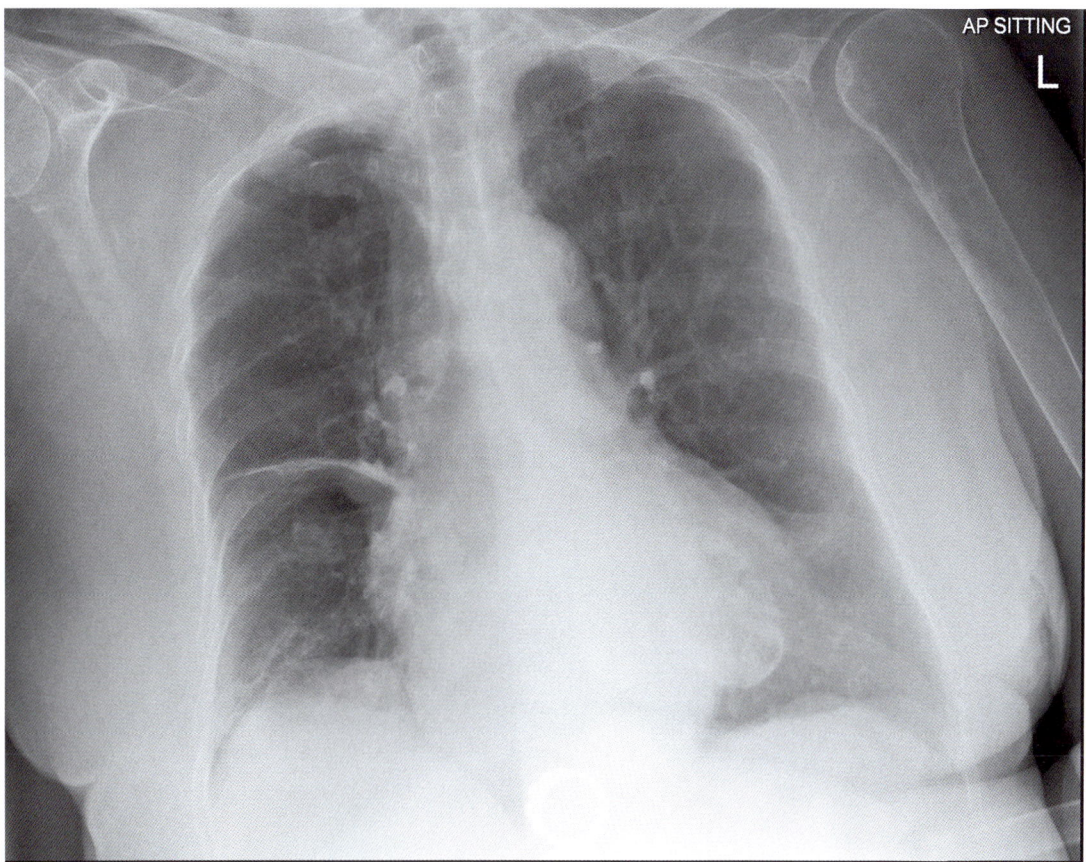

Figure 12.100

Answer to Case 60

Some fluid remains within the middle fissure but no further consolidation or collapse is demonstrated. What is interesting about this case is the calcified ventricular aneurysm, which was long-standing, and you can see it overlying the left heart border.

References and further reading

Armstrong, P. & Wastie, L. (1989). 'The Respiratory System and The Heart'. In: P. Armstrong & L. Wastie (eds) *Diagnostic Imaging*. 2nd edn. Oxford: Blackwell Scientific Publications. 12–116.

Bastos, R., Calhoon, J.H. & Baisden, C.E. (2008). Flail chest and pulmonary contusion. *Seminars in Thoracic and Cardiovascular Surgery*. **20**(1), 39–45.

Becher, R.P., Colonna, A.L. & Weaver, A.A. (2012). An innovative approach to predict the development of ARDS in patients with blunt trauma. *Journal of Trauma and Acute Care Surgery*. **73**(5), 129–35.

Binnay, C., Califf, R.M. & Hasselblad, V. (2005). Evaluation study of congestive heart failure and pulmonary artery catheterisation effectiveness: The ESCAPE trial. *Journal of the American Medical Association*. **294**, 1625–33.

Broder, J.S. (2011). *Diagnostic Imaging for the Emergency Physician*. Philadelphia: Elsevier Saunders. 297–372.

Brooks, A., Mahoney, P.F. & Hodgetts, T.J. (2007). *Major Trauma*. Edinburgh: Churchill Livingstone.

Buttaravoli, P. & Leffler, S.M. (2012). *Minor Emergencies*. 3rd edn. Elsevier. 236–39.

Channey, J.M., Edmond, M. & Plouder, M. (2012). Patients with rib fractures do not develop delayed pneumonia: a prospective multicenter cohort study of minor thoracic trauma. *Annals of Emergency Medicine*. **60**(6), 726–31.

Chapman, S. & Nakielny, S. (1992). 'The Respiratory Tract and the Cardiovascular System'. In: S. Chapman & S. Nakielny (eds) *Aids to Radiological Differential Diagnosis*. 3rd edn. London: W.B Saunders Co Ltd, 106–94.

Chen, J.T. (1997). *Essentials of Cardiac Imaging*. 2nd edn. Philadelphia: Lippincott-Raven.

Collins, J. & Stern, E. (2008). *Chest Radiology: The essentials*. 2nd edn. Philadelphia: Lippincott Williams & Wilkins.

Comstock, G.W. (2000). 'Epidemiology of tuberculosis'. In: L.B. Reichman & E.S. Hershfield (eds) *Tuberculosis: a comprehensive international approach*. 2nd edn. New York: Marcel Dekker. 129–56.

Cooper, J.M. & Kay, G.N. (2008). 'Basic concepts of pacing'. In: K.A. Ellenbogen & M.A. Wood (eds) *Cardiac Pacing & ICDs*. 5th edn. Oxford: Blackwell Publishing.

Corne, J., Carroll, M., Brown, I. & Delaney, D. (1997). *Chest X-ray Made Easy*. 2nd edn. Edinburgh: Churchill Livingstone.

Cottin, V. (2005). *Combined pulmonary fibrosis and emphysema: a distinct underrecognised entity.* https://erj.ersjournals.com/content/26/4/586 (Last accessed 7.7.2019).

Das, D. & Howett, D. (2009). *Chest Radiology: the essentials*. 2nd edn. Philadelphia: Lippincott Williams & Wilkins.

Davies, H., Gordon, I., Matthew, D.J., Helms, P., Kenney, I.J., Lutkin, J.E. & Lenney, W. (1990). Long-term follow-up after inhalation of foreign bodies. *Archives of Disease in Childhood*. **65/6**(619–21), 1468–2044.

De Lacey, G., Morley, S. & Berman, L. (2008). *The Chest X-ray: A Survival Guide*. London: Elsevier Saunders.

Devereux, G. (2007). *ABC of COPD*. Massachusetts: Blackwell Publishing.

Edey, A.J. & Hansell, D.M. (2009). CT lung cancer screening in the UK-NCBI. *British Journal of Radiology*. **82**(979), 529–31.

El Fatih, I.M. (1995). 'Tuberculosis in the adult'. In: L. Lutwick (ed.) *Tuberculosis – A clinical handbook*. Chapman and Hall Medical. 20–53.

Ellis, S. (2010). *Interpreting Chest X-rays*. Banbury: Scion Publishing.

Ellis, S. & Flower, C. (2006). *The WHO Manual of Diagnostic Imaging: Radiographic Anatomy and Interpretation of the Chest and Pulmonary System*. Published by the World Health Organisation in collaboration with the International Society of Radiology.

Feigen, D. (2010). Lateral chest radiography: a systematic approach. *Academic Radiology*. **17**(12) 1560–66.

Felson, B. (1973a). 'Localisation of intrathoracic lesions'. In: B. Felson (ed.) *Chest Roentgenology*. London: WB Saunders. 22–70.

Felson, B. (1973b). 'The Lobes' In: B. Felson (ed.) *Chest Roentgenology*. London: WB Saunders. 71–142.

Felson, B. & Felson, H. (1950). Localisation of intrathoracic lesions by means of the posterior-anterior roentgenogram: The silhouette sign. *Radiology*. **55**, 363–74.

Finfer, S. & Delaney, A. (2006). Pulmonary artery catheters. *British Medical Journal*. **333**, 930–31.

Gleeson, F.V. (2006). The chest radiograph in heart disease. *Medicine*. **34**(4), 136–41.

Goodman, R. (2007). *Felson's Principles of Chest Roentgenology, a Programmed Text*. 3rd edn. Philadelphia: Elsevier Saunders.

Greaves, I., Porter, K.M. & Ryan, J.M. (eds) (2001). *Trauma Care Manual*. London: Arnold.

Grenier, P. (2001). 'Chronic airflow obstruction'. In: R.G. Grainger, D.J. Allison, A. Adam & A.K. Dixon (eds) *Diagnostic Radiology: a textbook of medical imaging*. 4th edn. London: Churchill Livingstone. 453–61.

Hammond, J.M., Potgieterer, P.D., Linton, D.M. & Forder, A.A. (1991). Intensive care management of community acquired Klebsiella pneumonia. *Respiratory Medicine.* **85/1**(11–16), 0954–6111.

Hansell, D., Armstrong, P., Lynch, D. & McAdams, H. (2005). *Imaging Diseases of the Chest.* 4th edn. Phildelphia: Elsevier Mosby.

Hartnell, G.G. & Raphael, M.J. (2001). 'Cardiac anatomy and enlargement'. In: R.G. Grainger, D.J. Allison, A. Adam & A.K. Dixon (eds) *Diagnostic Radiology: a textbook of medical imaging.* 4th edn. London: Churchill Livingstone. 673–91.

Hogg, J.C. (2001). *Chronic obstructive pulmonary disease: an overview of pathology and pathogenesis.* https://www.ncbi.nlm.nih.gov/pubmed/11199102 (Last accessed 7.7.2019).

Hollman, A.S. & Adams, F.G. (1989). The influence of the lordotic projection on the interpretation of the chest radiograph. *Clinical Radiology.* **40**, 360–64.

Hunt, I., Muers, M. & Treasure, T. (2009). *ABC of Lung Cancer.* Philadelphia: Wiley-Blackwell and Sow Ltd.

Ida, M. (1995). 'Epidemiology of Tuberculosis'. In: L. Lutwick (ed.) *Tuberculosis – a clinical handbook.* Chapman and Hall Medical. 20–53

Karthik, S. (March 2013). *Lecture and Quiz on Tubes and Lines: Chest Reporting for Trainee Radiologists.* Radiology Teaching Academy, Leeds General Infirmary.

Katz, R. (2012). *Basic Chest Interpretation Programme 2.* http://www.askdoctorclarke.com (Last accessed 7.7.2019).

Kaul, S. (2007). *Managing chronic obstructive pulmonary disease.* Wiley online books. https://onlinelibrary.wiley.com/doi/10.1002/9780470697603.ch1 (Last accessed 7.7.2019).

Kazerooni, E.A. (2001). *High resolution CT of the lungs.* NCBI. https://www.ncbi.nlm.nih.gov/pubmed/11517038 (Last accessed 7.7.2019).

Kerley, P. (1933). Radiology in heart disease. *British Medical Journal* 2. 594–97. Cited in: Hansell, D., Armstrong, P., Lynch, D. & McAdams, H. (2005). *Imaging Diseases of the Chest.* 4th edn. Philadelphia: Elsevier Mosby.

Ketai, L., Lofrgren, R. & Meholic, J. (2006). 'Pulmonary Neoplasm'. In: L. Ketai, R. Lofrgren & J. Meholic (eds). *Fundamentals of Chest Radiology.* 2nd edn. Philadelphia: Elsevier Saunders. 140–58.

Malagari, K. & Roussos, C. (2001). 'Chest trauma'. In: M. Sperber (ed) *Radiologic Diagnosis of Chest Disease.* 2nd edn. London: Springer-Verlag.

Manser, R., Irving, L., Stone, C., Boynes, G. & Abramson, M. (2009). Screening for Lung Cancer. *Cochrane Database of Systematic Reviews,* Issue 1.

Mettler, F. (1996). 'Chest'. In: F. Mettler (ed). *Essentials of Radiology.* London: Saunders. 43–114.

Miller, S. (1997). 'Cardiac Imaging'. In: Weissleder, R., Rieumont, M. & Wittenberg (eds). *Primer of Diagnostic Imaging.* 2nd edn. London: Mosby. 100–49.

Moses, H.W., Miller, B.D., Moulton, K.P. & Schneider, J.A. (2000). *A Practical Guide to Cardiac Pacing.* 2nd edn. Chichester: Wiley Blackwell.

National Heart, Lung and Blood Institute Acute Respiratory Distress Syndrome (ARDS) Clinical Trials Network (2006). Pulmonary-artery versus central venous catheter to guide treatment of acute lung injury. *New England Journal of Medicine.* **354**, 2213–73.

Neragi-Miandoab, S. (2006). Malignant pleural effusion, current and evolving approaches for its diagnosis and management. *Lung Cancer.* 54(1), 1–9.

NHS National Patient Safety Agency (2011). *Reducing the harm caused by misplaced nasogastric feeding tubes in adults, children and infants.* NPSA/2011/PSA002.

NICE guidelines (2005). *The diagnosis and treatment of lung cancer* (update). https://www.ncbi.nlm.nih.gov/pubmed/15835336 (Last accessed 7.7.2019).

NICE guidelines (2011). *Lung cancer: diagnosis and management.* https://www.nice.org.uk/guidance/cg121 (Last accessed 7.7.2019).

Nowak ,T.J. & Handford, A.G. (1999). *Essentials of Pathophysiology: Concepts and Applications for the Health Care Professions.* 2nd edn. Boston: McGraw-Hill.

Oktay, A. (2011). *Signs in Chest Imaging – Diagnostic and Interventional Radiology.* 17, 18–29.

Ormerod, L. (1998). 'Respiratory Tuberculosis'. In: P. Davies (ed.) *Clinical Tuberculosis.* 2nd edn. Chapman and Hall. 155–74.

Pass, H. & Carbone, D. (2005). *Principles and Practice of Lung Cancer, the official reference text of IASLL.* Philadelphia: Wolters Kluwer/Lippincott, Williams and Wilkins.

Piessens, W.F. & Nardell, E.A. (2000). 'Pathogenesis of tuberculosis'. In: L.B. Reichman & E.S. Hershfield (eds) *Tuberculosis: a comprehensive international approach.* 2nd edn. London: Springer. 180–92.

Pressley, C.M., Fry, W.R., Philips, A.S. & Berry, S.D. (2012). Predicting outcome of patients with chest wall injury. *American Journal of Surgery.* **204**(6), 910–13.

Reed, J.C. (2003). *Chest Radiology: Plain Film Patterns and Differential Diagnosis.* 5th edn. Philadelphia: Mosby.

Reuter, M. (1996). Review article. Trauma of the chest. *European Journal of Radiology.* **6**, 707–16.

Rojanapithayakorn, W. & Nari, J. (1999). *Tuberculosis and HIV, some questions and answers.* World Health Organisation, Regional office for South East Asia, New Delhi, India.

Royal College of Radiologists (2012). *Standards of practice and guidance for trauma radiology in severely injured patients.* http://www.rcr.ac.uk/system/files/publication/field_publication_files/bfcr155_traumaradiol.pdf (Last accessed 7.7.2019).

Schnyder, P. & Wintermark, M. (2000). *Radiology of Blunt Trauma of the Chest.* Berlin: Springer-Verlag.

Shure, D. (2006). Pulmonary artery catheters – peace at last? *New England Journal of Medicine.* **354**, 2273.

Steiner, G.M. (1993a). 'The Respiratory Tract'. In: G.M. Steiner (ed.) *Essential Paediatric Radiology.* Oxford: Blackwell Scientific Publications. 129–56.

Steiner, G.M. (1993b). 'The Heart'. In: G.M. Steiner (ed.) *Essential Paediatric Radiology.* Oxford: Blackwell Scientific Publications. 157–76.

Sunderamoorthy, D., Ahuja, S., Grant, A. & Mian, T. (2005). Right upper lobe consolidation: an unusual complication of an uneventful endotracheal intubation. *Emergency Medicine Journal.* **22/9**(669–70),1472–0213.

Sutton, D. ed (2003). *Textbook of Radiology and Imaging.* 7th edn. Edinburgh: Churchill Livingstone.

Tortora, G. & Anagnostakos, N. (1990a). 'The respiratory system'. In: G. Tortora & N. Anagnostakos (eds) *Principles of Anatomy and Physiology.* 6th edn. New York: Harper and Row. 689–730.

Tortora, G. & Anagnostakos, N. (1990b). 'The cardiovascular system, the heart, vessels and routes'. In: G. Tortora & N. Anagnostakos (eds) *Principles of Anatomy and Physiology.* 6th edn. New York: Harper and Row. 572–653.

Watson J. (2013). *TB in the UK: 2013 report.* https://assets.publishing.service.gov.uk/government/uploads/system/uploads/attachment_data/file/325632/TB_in_the_UK.pdf (Last accessed 7.7.2019).

Weaver, A.A., Danelson, K.A., Armstrong, E.G., Hoth, J.J. & Stitzel, J.D. (2013). Investigation of pulmonary contusion extent and its correlation to crash, occupant and injury characteristics in motor vehicle crashes. *Accident Analysis and Prevention.* **50**, 223–33.

Weissleder, R., Rieumont, M. & Wittenberg, J. (1997). 'Chest Imaging'. In: R. Weissleder, M. Rieumont & J. Wittenberg (eds) *Primer of Diagnostic Imaging.* 2nd edn. London: Mosby. 1–99.

Whitson, B.A., McGonigal, M.D., Anderson, C.P. & Dries, D.J. (2013). Increasing number of rib fractures do not worsen outcome: an analysis of the national trauma data. *The American Surgeon.* 1555–9823, **79**(2), 140–50.

Wiwat, R. (1999). *The global plan to stop tuberculosis.* https://www.opensocietyfoundations.org/uploads/9842fd1c-8dea-4f0d-a1e5-1d633ac64fef/tb_complete.pdf (Last accessed 7.7.2019).

Wood, M.K. & Spiro, S.G. (2001). 'Carcinoma of the lung'. In: M. Sperber (ed.) *Radiologic Diagnosis of Chest Disease.* 2nd edn. London: Springer-Verlag. 424–40.

World Health Organisation Report (2011). *Global Tuberculosis Control 2011.* WHO.

Zhao, Y.R. (2011). *NELSON lung cancer screening study – NCBI.* http://www.ncbi.nlm.nih.gov/pmc/articles/PMC3266562/ (Last accessed 7.7.2019).

Zylak, C.J., Littleton, J.T. & Durizch, M.L. (1988). Illusory consolidation of the left lower lobe: a pitfall of portable radiography. *Radiology.* **167**, 653–55.

Index

ABCDEF method 13
acquired immune deficiency syndrome (AIDS) 69
adult respiratory distress syndrome (ARDS) 152
air bronchograms 19
alveolar oedema 30
aortic aneurysm 134
aortic incompetence 31
aortic rupture 53
aortic stenosis 31
artefacts 94, 100
asbestosis 65, 66
asthma 68
atelectasis 46
automated implantable cardioverter defibrillator (AICD) 108
azygos fissure 96
azygos lobe 84

benign appearances 25
bronchiectasis 21, 150
bronchial carcinoid 45
bronchial obstruction 21
bullae 67, 92, 164

cardiac failure, see heart failure
cardiac trauma 54
cardiomegaly 182, 186
cardiothoracic ratio (CTR) 4, 27, 182
cardiovascular disorders 27
central venous pressure (CVP) line 59
cervical ribs 118
cervicothoracic sign 18
chamber dilation 27
chamber enlargement 28
chamber hypertrophy 27
chest anatomy 4
chest drain 89, 90
chest infection 96, 124, 174
chest trauma 49–54
chronic bronchitis 68
chronic cardiac failure (CCF) 142, 182
chronic obstructive pulmonary disease (COPD) 67, 170, 191
collagen vascular diseases 63
consolidation 19, 124
consolidation, patchy 20

dermatomyositis 64
diaphragm 2, 5, 10
diaphragm, rupture of the 54

emphysema 67
endotracheal (ET) tube 55

Felson, Ben 15, 18
fibrosis, determining the cause of 66
flail segment 50
fractures 50

granulomas 44

haemothorax 50, 98, 156
hamartoma 44
heart disease, signs of 27
heart failure 30, 86, 126, 188
heart size 4, 27
heart structures 5
hiatus hernia 84, 114, 130
hilar 8, 10
hilum convergence sign 17
hilum overlay sign 17, 18
humeral head dislocation 186
humeral head, fracture of the 180

idiopathic pulmonary fibrosis 63
inspiration, assessing 2
interstitial oedema 29
ischaemic heart disease 32

lateral chest x-ray 8, 9
laws of motion 49
left atrial myxoma 32
left lower lobe, collapse of the 22
lobar collapse 23, 24, 25, 82, 112, 132, 166, 168
lobar fibrosis 21
lobar pneumonia, causes 20
lung cancer 33, 78, 80, 132
lung cancer, clinical manifestations of 34
lung cancer investigations 36
lung collapse 82, 162
lung contusion 50, 53
lung nodules 43–47, 144, 146
lung tumour screening 39, 40

lung tumours, chest x-ray features of 34, 35
lung tumours, location and frequency of 33
lungs 6, 7
lymphangitis 35

mediastinal lines 7
metastases 136
mitral incompetence 31
mitral stenosis 31

nasoenteric tube 61
nasogastric (NG) tube 56, 57, 103, 104

osteophyte 138

PA/AP/supine x-rays 4
pacemakers 61, 62
Pancoast's tumours 34, 158
paratracheal stripe 7
paravertebral stripe displacement 7
pectus excavatum 110
pericardial disease 28
pericardial fat pad 128, 130
plasmacytoma 178
pleural drainage tube 60
pleural effusion 22, 156, 182
pleural plaque 116, 160
pneumoconiosis 65
pneumomediastinum 52, 53
pneumonia 46, 142
pneumothorax 22, 50, 51, 52, 59, 88, 89, 90, 102, 106, 118, 120, 122, 162, 172, 180, 194
polyarteritis nodosa 64
posterior anterior x-rays 1
pulmonary artery catheter 59, 60
pulmonary artery hypertension 29
pulmonary blood flow, increase or decrease 29
pulmonary collapse 20, 21, 22, 23
pulmonary embolus 22
pulmonary infarct 47
pulmonary nodules, causes of 43
pulmonary oedema 29
pulmonary venous hypertension 29
pulmonary vessels 28

radiation pneumonitis 63
relative absorption values of tissues 16
renal cancer 135
rheumatoid lung 64
rib fractures 50, 51, 98, 148, 156, 160, 184, 186, 194
ribs, counting 2
road traffic collision (RTC) 49, 50

S sign 132
sail sign 23
sarcoid 190
sarcoidosis 64, 65

sclerodermia 64
shoulder dislocation 114
silhouette sign 15, 16, 17, 18, 19, 21, 23, 82, 96, 133
skin fold 86
solitary metastasis 46
supine patient 3
Swan-Ganz catheter 59, 60
systemic lupus erythematosus 64

thoracoabdominal sign 18
TNM staging system 37
tracheo-bronchial rupture 53

tracheostomy tube 61
tricuspid stenosis and incompetence 31
tuberculosis (TB) 69–73, 140, 154, 172
tuberculosis, active 71, 72
tuberculosis, miliary 172
tuberculosis, post-primary 70
tuberculosis, primary 70

valvular heart disease 31

Wegener's granulomatosis 64

x-rays, quality issues 2, 3